Surgical Management of Head and Neck Pathologies

Edited by Ho-Hyun (Brian) Sun

Published in London, United Kingdom

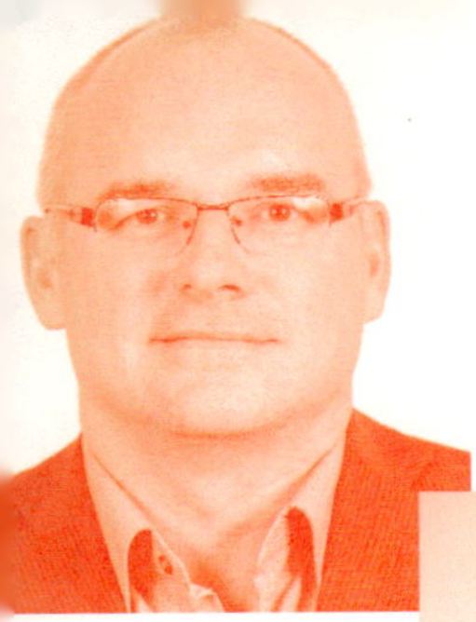
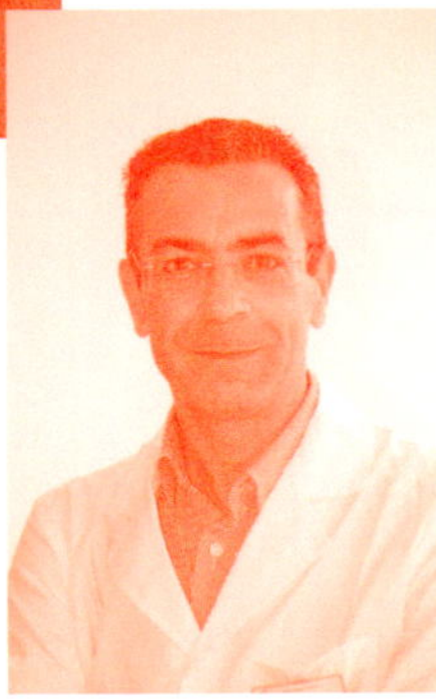
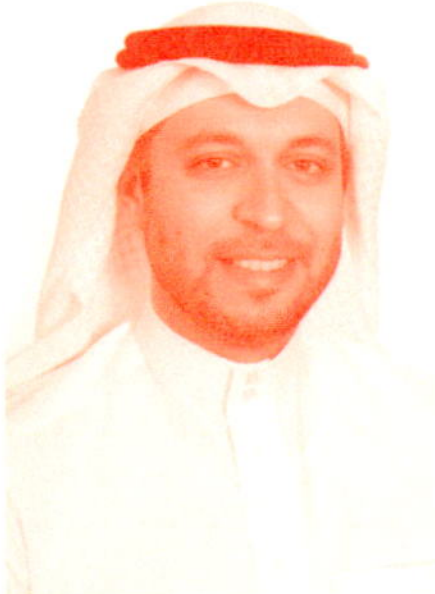
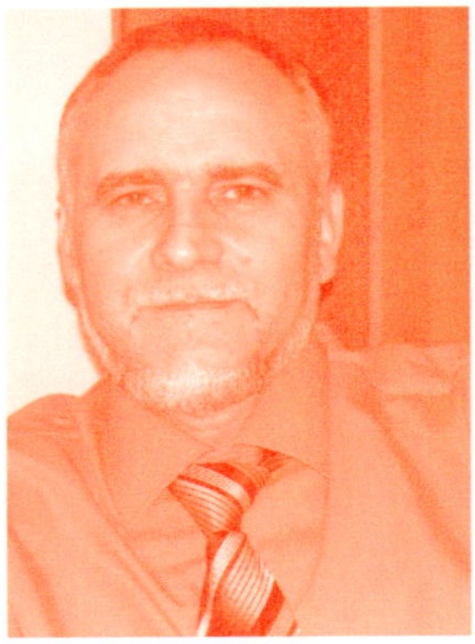
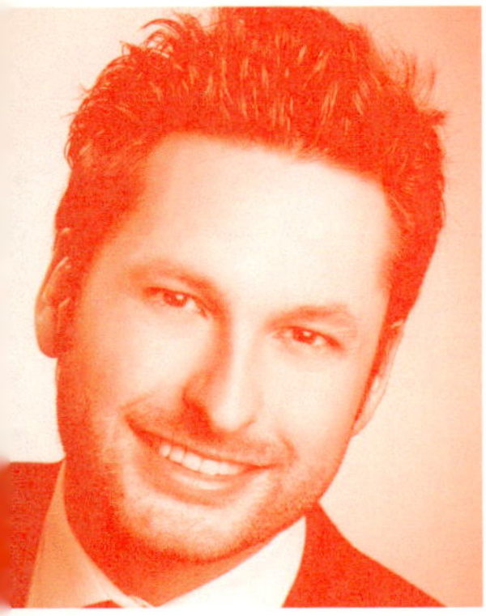
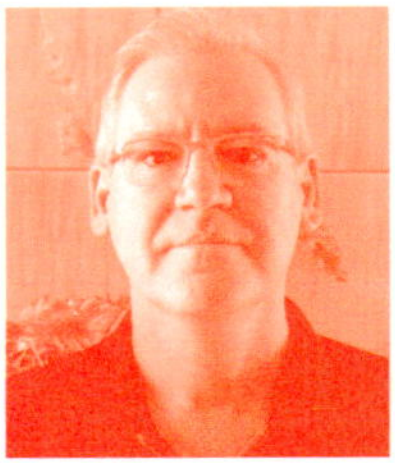
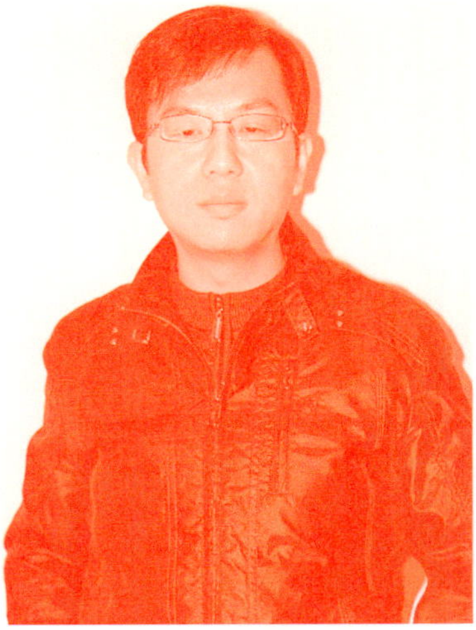

IntechOpen

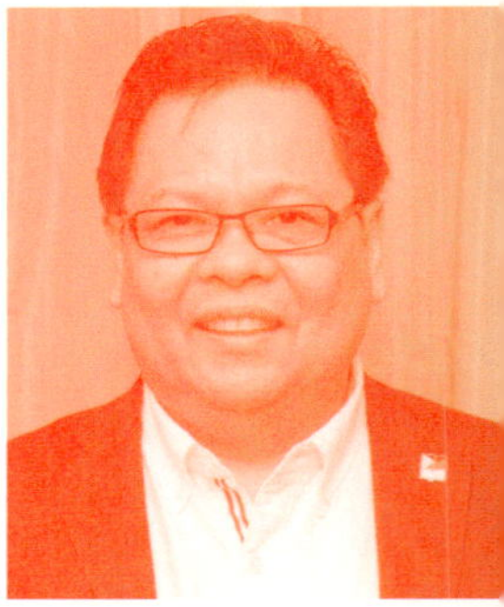
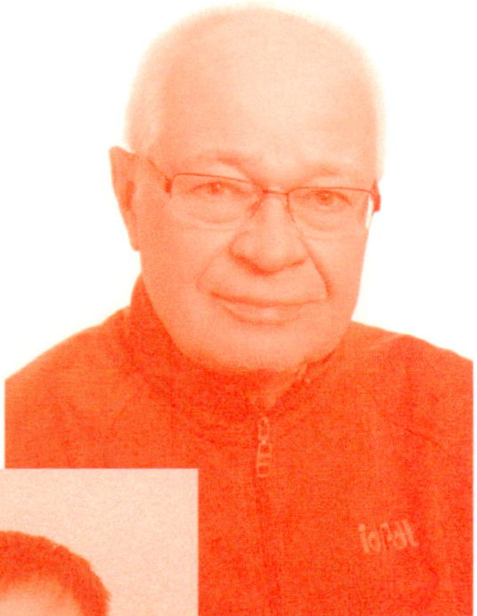
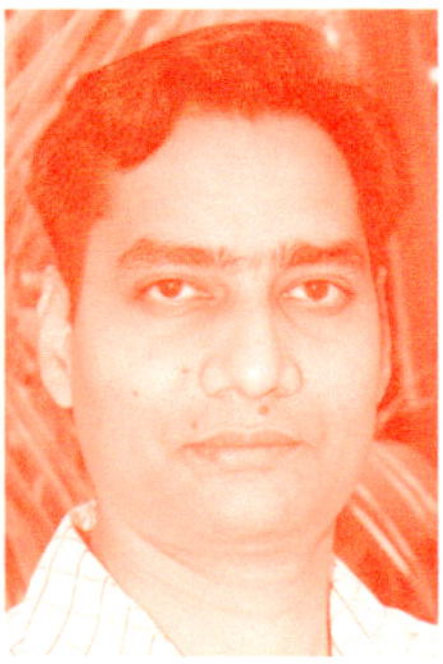
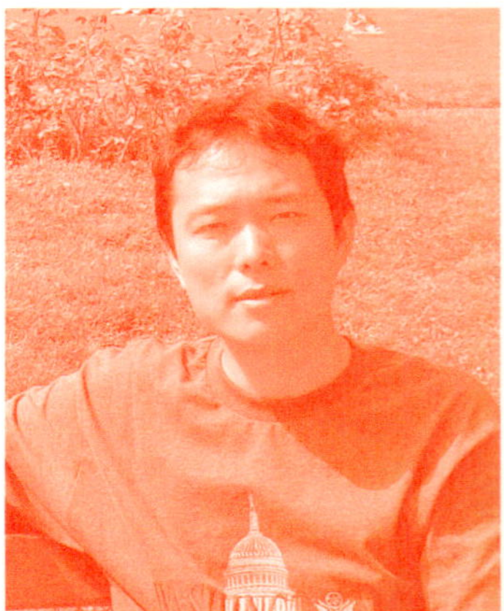
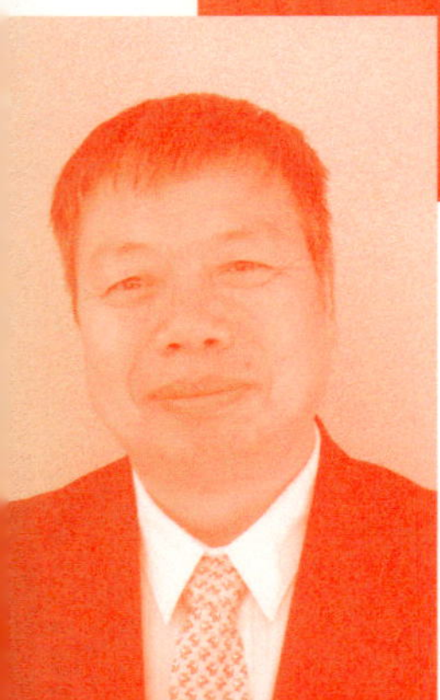
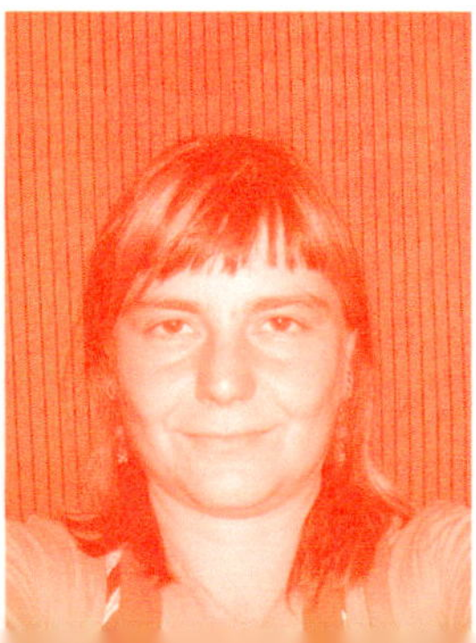

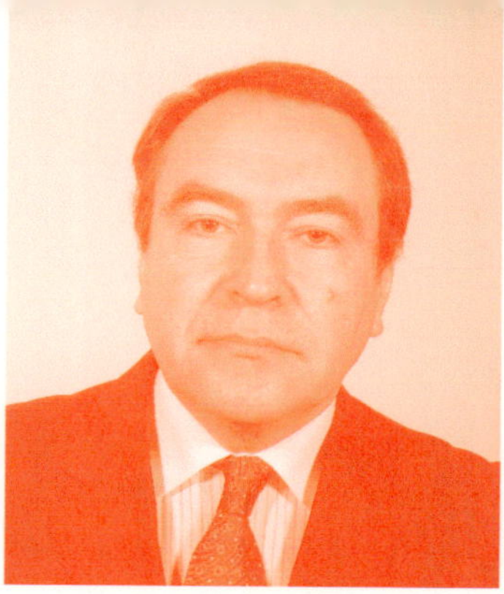

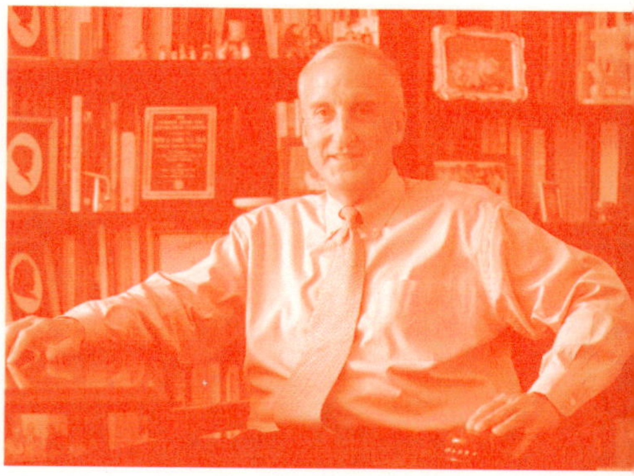

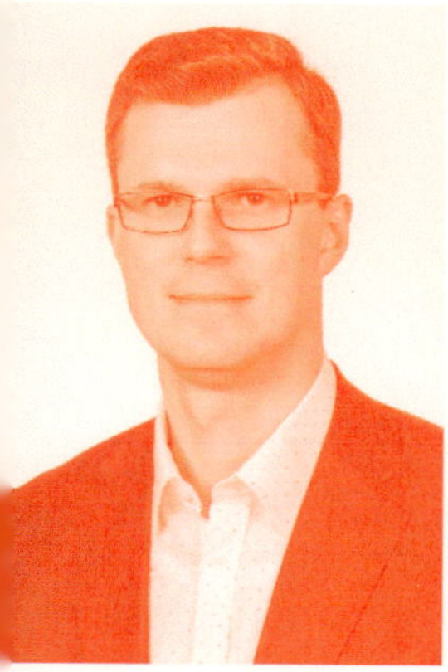

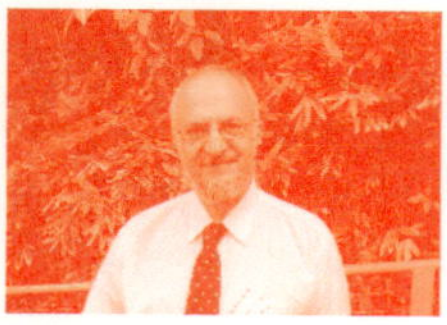

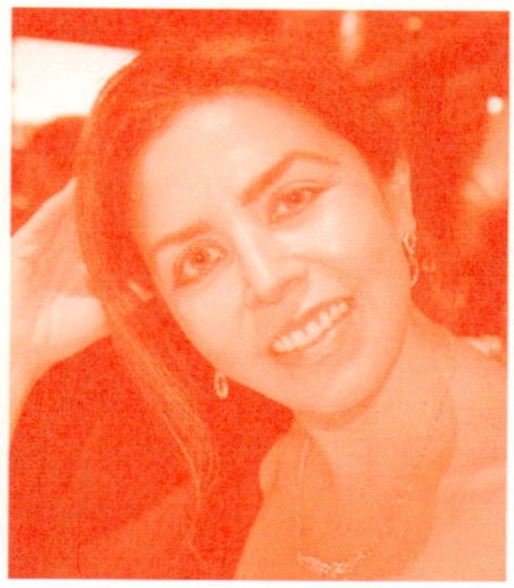

Supporting open minds since 2005

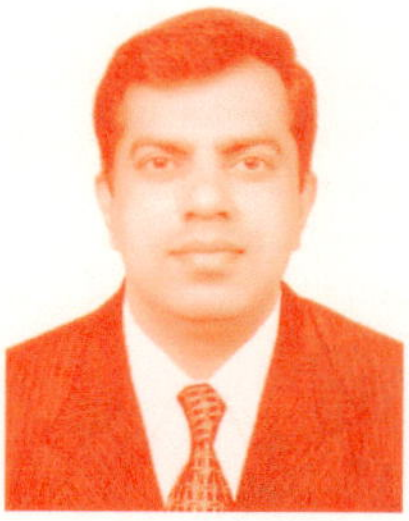

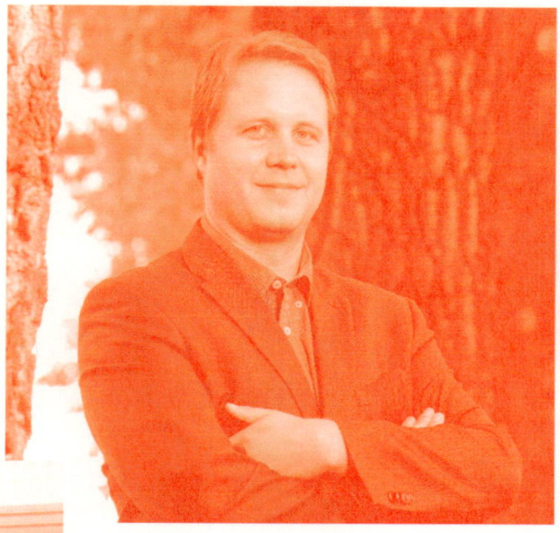

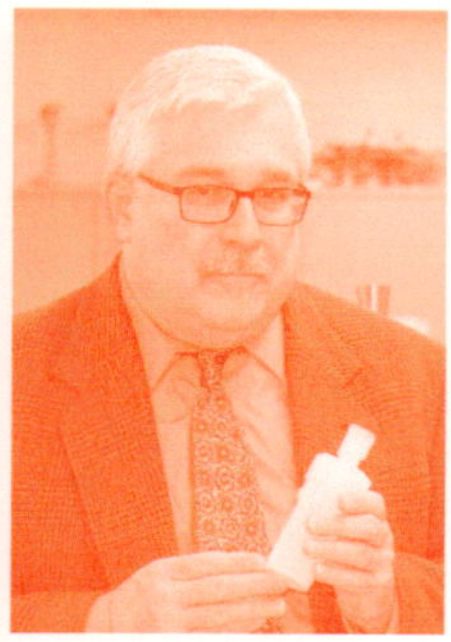

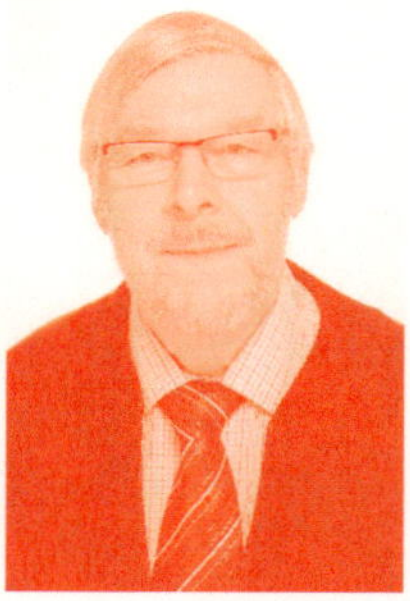

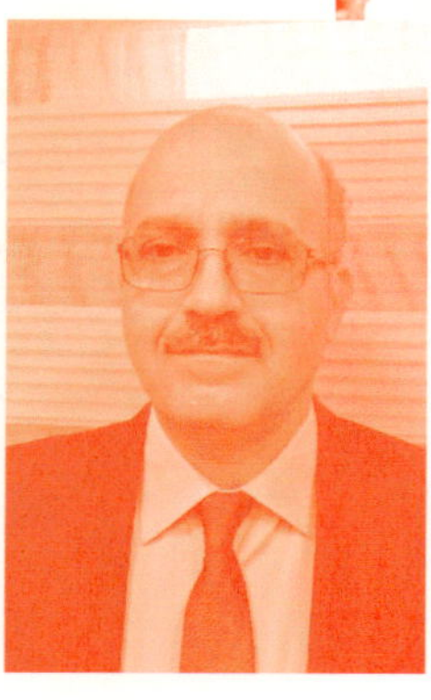

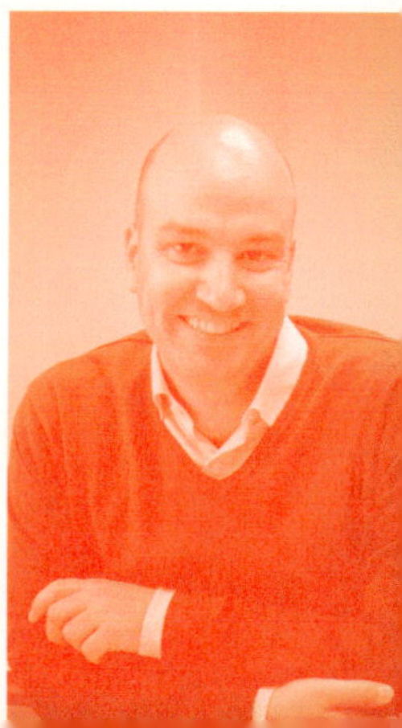

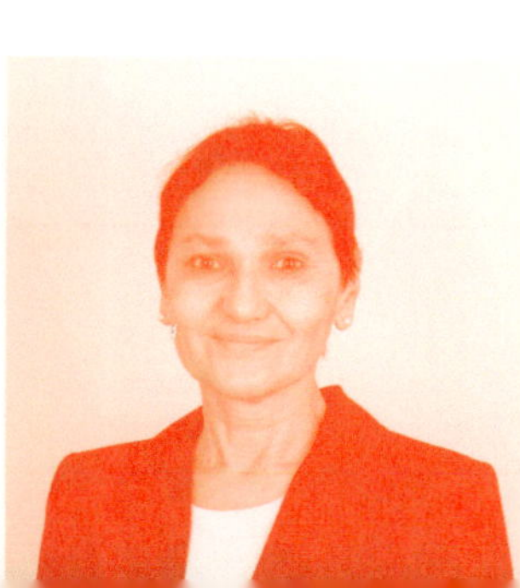

Surgical Management of Head and Neck Pathologies
http://dx.doi.org/10.5772/intechopen.87598
Edited by Ho-Hyun (Brian) Sun

Contributors
Amalia Raluca Ceausu, Anca Maria Cimpean, Marius Raica, Eugen Radu Boia, Eugen Sorin Boia, Bruce Ashford, Takako Eva Yabe, Ho-Hyun (Brian) Sun, Sally Sun, Muhammad Jaffar Khan, Tarek Tageldin, Muhammad Waqas Farooqi, Odai Qasim Khamash, Umair Shahid, Mohamed El-Fatih Abdul-Rahman, Mohamed El-Arref, Jazib Hassan, Nguyen Pham, Isabella Rodoni, Manish Anand, Shreya Panwar, Guillermo Plaza, Juan Manuel Maza-Solano, Pablo Parente, Juan Carlos Amor-Dorado, Christian Calvo-Henriquez, Kris R. Jatana, Dustin A. Silverman, Ross Wanner, Patrick Walz, Matthew O. Old

First published in London, United Kingdom, 2021 by IntechOpen
IntechOpen is the global imprint of INTECHOPEN LIMITED, registered in England and Wales, registration number: 11086078, 5 Princes Gate Court, London, SW7 2QJ, United Kingdom
Printed in Croatia

British Library Cataloguing-in-Publication Data
A catalogue record for this book is available from the British Library

Additional hard and PDF copies can be obtained from orders@intechopen.com

Surgical Management of Head and Neck Pathologies
Edited by Ho-Hyun (Brian) Sun
p. cm.
Print ISBN 978-1-83881-983-5
Online ISBN 978-1-83881-984-2
eBook (PDF) ISBN 978-1-83881-985-9

For EU product safety concerns:
IN TECH d.o.o., Prolaz Marije Krucifikse Kozulić 3, 51000 Rijeka, Croatia, info@intechopen.com or visit our website at intechopen.com.

Meet the editor

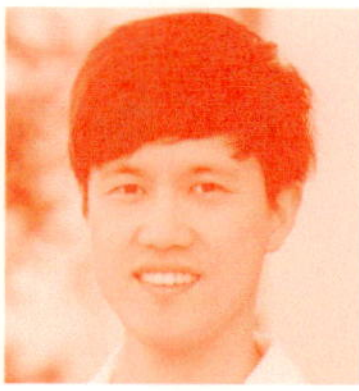

Ho-Hyun (Brian) Sun, DMD, MS, is an oral and maxillofacial surgeon, a clinical assistant professor at the Western University of Health Sciences, California, a clinical instructor at the Department of Oral and Maxillofacial Surgery, University of the Pacific, California, and a graduate alumnus of the UCLA Center for Oral/Head and Neck Oncology Research. His areas of interest include dentoalveolar surgery, orthognathic surgery, sleep surgery, trauma, pathology, and anesthesiology. He has numerous publications in journals, textbooks, and reference books to his credit. He is a lifelong clinician, researcher, and educator with interests not only in the clinical but also in the scientific aspects of surgery. Dr. Sun is comfortable with both teaching and researching maxillofacial biology.

Contents

Preface

Because of compact architecture, proximity to vital structures, and critical esthetic components, surgical treatments of the head and neck require extensive considerations. Several modern paradigms in soft tissue and osseous surgeries have led to significant improvements since the earlier days of surgery.

As scientists, we surgeons strive to "improve on the improvements" towards bettering the lives of our patients even further. This textbook was envisioned not only as an overview of some of the pre-existing tenets of the head, maxillofacial, and neck surgery but also to introduce new ideas from colleagues all around the world.

To that end, we begin with a vision towards molecular classifications of squamous carcinoma, which has largely eluded our quest for personalized cures. We then discuss the oft-overlooked field of pediatric malignancies, followed by two chapters exploring pre-existing neck and maxillofacial reconstruction techniques. Subsequent chapters discuss airway management, whether during anesthesia for the surgery of acquired lesions, during patients' daily sleep regimes, or in those with congenital airway defects. We end the volume with a chapter on the new challenge of COVID-19, which threatens not only our health but also the current healthcare infrastructure.

Our goal is to introduce concepts that are both novel and proven. International cooperation was made to help ensure that a wide range of perspectives is presented. To this end, we thank our dear authors across the globe who have invested heavily to provide both creativity and the burden of proof.

We hope readers enjoy this book as much as we enjoyed preparing it. Thank you for taking the time to read our work.

Ho-Hyun (Brian) Sun, DMD, MS
Clinical Instructor,
University of the Pacific,
California, USA

Clinical Assistant Professor,
Western University of Health Sciences,
California, USA

Surgeon,
Bay Area Oral Surgery Management,
California, USA

Section 1

Overview of Pathologic Classifications

Chapter 1

Toward a Molecular Classification of the Head and Neck Squamous Cell Carcinoma

Amalia Raluca Ceausu, Eugen Radu Boia, Eugen Sorin Boia, Anca Maria Cimpean and Marius Raica

Abstract

The frequency of the squamous cell carcinoma of the head and neck is constantly increasing, with over 550.000 new cases registered globally each year. The conventional histopathological diagnosis most commonly indicates the squamous cell carcinoma as tumor type and G2 as differentiation grade. Despite of this relative morphological uniformity, there is a great heterogeneity in the molecular profile, the therapeutic response and prognosis. Most probably, this entity includes many diseases, similar in basic morphologic features, but different in the biological behavior. Trying to answer this question and to show discrepancies when they exist, we have evaluated in this book chapter, our own results and data from the literature in terms of molecular profile at the protein level, including the spectrum of proliferation markers, growth factors and their receptors, stromal proliferation, angiogenesis and lymphangiogenesis. These data will allow to identify some major criteria for a better stratification of cases, selected for gene analysis and personalized therapy as a future perspective and direction.

Keywords: HNSCC, molecular profile, stroma, stratification of cases, gene analysis

1. Introduction

The recent data regarding the global cancer statistic [1] indicate an increase number of new diagnosed HNSCC cases each year. Despite the efforts, the 5 years OS rate of HNSCC has not improve significantly over the last years. There are several reasons that can be mentioned: the classic causative factors such as alcohol consumption and tobacco usage, the presence of the lymph nodes metastases at the time of the diagnosis, important increase in the HPV infections in the Western world [2]. Between 40 to 60% of HNSCC treated patients have recurrence and not respond to subsequent therapeutic interventions [3]. Another important reason may be the accentuated heterogeneity of HNSCC at the molecular level, the inability of a clear stratification of the cases and the absence of a certain link between the molecular subtypes and the clinical outcome. A number between four and six molecular types of HNSCC were described in the literature. Chung [4] described four distinct subtypes: first (displays EGFR pathway and hypoxia related molecular signatures), the second is mesenchymal marker enriched, the third has features of normal epithelia and the fourth expresses high levels of transcripts coding for antioxidant and detoxification enzymes. The four groups of HNSCC proposed by Walter [5] are: basal, mesenchymal, atypical, and classical. Five subgroups of HNSCC were described also by another research team: three HPV negative (basal, classical non- HPV and mesenchymal non -HPV) and two HPV positive (classical HPV and mesenchymal HPV) [6]. Other author described six subtypes (immunoreactive, inflammatory, HPV-like, classical, hypoxia associated and mesenchymal) [7]. The heterogeneity of the tumor microenvironment and the clear histological margin used today may be other reasons for tumor recurrences.

We try in the following to identify some major criteria for a better stratification of the cases, and for a better surveillance of the postoperative margins, targeting the personalized therapy.

2. The conventional histopathological diagnostic and morphological features

The head and neck squamous cell carcinomas are epithelial tumors originating in the covering mucosa of oral cavity, larynx, oropharynx, and hypopharynx [8]. In an attempt to cover the heterogeneous spectrum of these tumors, the most used clinical management is based on anatomic location, phenotype, evaluation of the existence of tumor -node-metastasis by the TNM classification and the depth of tumor invasions [9]. The WHO classification of head and neck tumors includes tumors of the nasal cavity, paranasal sinuses and skull base (with the keratinizing, non-keratinizing and spindle cell squamous cell carcinoma types), tumors of the nasopharynx, of the hypopharynx, larynx, trachea, parapharyngeal space (with the conventional, verrucous, basaloid, papillary, spindle cell types of squamous cell carcinomas), tumors of the oral cavity and mobile tongue, of the oropharynx (base of the tongue, tonsils, adenoids) with HPV positive and HPV negative types of squamous cell carcinoma, tumors and tumors-like lesions of the neck and lymph nodes, tumors of salivary glands, odontogenic and maxillofacial bone tumors, tumors of the ear and paraganglion tumors [10].

In the conventional histopathological diagnosis, the squamous cell carcinoma may be graded as well, moderate, and poorly differentiated type. The well differentiated type of keratinized squamous cell carcinoma is characterized by the presence of the keratinizing and para-keratinizing pearls. Morphological features in the moderately differentiated squamous cell carcinoma are nuclear pleomorphism, mitoses, including atypical type and less keratinization. The poorly differentiated type is characterized by the predominance of the immature cells, a high number of typical and atypical mitoses, reduced keratinization and necrosis either over large areas of the section or in the center of the tumor areas, variable in extent. Most HNSCC are moderately- differentiated [11, 12] aspect sustained by our data where a percentage of 73.8% and 71% from HNSCC evaluated cases were diagnosed as G2 [13, 14]. The non-keratinized squamous cell carcinomas have the following morphological features: the existence of a large, interconnected band of tumor epithelial cells without keratinization and minimal or absent necrosis, pleomorphic cells, hyperchromasia and an intense mitotic activity.

The histologic grade prognostic impact remains controversial in HNSCC. It was accepted by the current edition of the Classification of Head and Neck Tumors but with the mention that grading alone does not correlate well with prognosis [15]. It is not a part of the UICC staging system, but some data consider high grade as an indication for the adjuvant treatment in OSCC [16, 17].

Starting from these premises it may be launched the question why the patients with the same histological grade have such a heterogeneous therapeutic response and prognosis.

3. The molecular profile at the protein level- cytokeratins, vimentin, podoplanin

The present molecular classification described four types of HNSCC as following: classical, basal, mesenchymal, and atypical subgroups. Excepted from this are the hypopharyngeal cancers characterized by the absence of the BA subgroup.

Keratins are a family of the intermediate filament proteins which are present in epithelial cells. Some of the main functions of keratins are structural in forming the cytoskeleton, protein synthesis, cell growth, signaling, organelle transport, mobility, and cell proliferation [18]. The keratin pattern distribution in a stratified epithelium is as follows: K1, 2, 10 and 11 are positive in cornified cells, K4 and 13 in stratified cells and K5 and 14 in basal cells [19].

The aberrant expression of keratins was found to be associated with HNSCC development and progression. High values of K 8, 17 and 19 immunoexpression were noticed in the biopsies of head and neck squamous cell carcinoma patients [20].

Keratin 5 was showed to be expressed with value of score between 1 and 3 (more than 30% positive cells), in squamous cell carcinoma with different histological grade and anatomical localization [21]. K5 together with EGFR, p63, CD 117 may be a helpful marker for define a distinct class of HNSCC (basal -like type, characterized by K5+/EGFR +/p63+/CD117+ profile). On the other hand, keratin 5 expression has been shown to correlate with the intermediate phenotype of cells involved in the epithelial-mesenchymal transition phenomenon [13, 22]. Some data demonstrated the by the immunohistochemical evaluation a loss of epithelial markers such as keratin 76 and epithelial cell adhesion molecule in the HNSCC [23, 24]. E- cadherin, involved in the cancer progression and metastasis by decrease of cellular adhesion and increase in cellular motility is co-expressed with Ep CAM. A decrease of E-cadherin expression associated with HPV 18 positivity were found in well and moderately differentiated type of HNSCC with larynx, oropharynx, pharyngo- laryngeal, and nasal-sinus localization. The rhino-pharynx, hypo-pharyngeal and laryngeal HPV18 negative cases were associated with a decrease of E-cadherin values in the moderately, poorly, and undifferentiated types.

The demonstrated role of cytokeratins in the diagnosis and prognosis of squamous cell carcinomas by using surrogate markers and biopsy tissues, oriented the research in the direction of a non-invasive diagnostic biomarker such as salivary keratins for the HNSCC [14, 19, 25].

The other molecule expressed in the basal cells of stratified epithelium is K14 which has an important role in cell differentiation. It was shown that K14 downregulation is associated with an increase in TAp63 and Notch-1 intracellular expression which regulates genes responsible for differentiation [26].

Vimentin is an intermediate filament intensely expressed in cells with mesenchymal phenotype. Its expression in oral epithelial cells has been linked by the tumor invasion, metastasis and EMT phenomenon [27].

It was shown that miR-876-5p, a tumor suppressor in HNSCC, represent a novel therapeutic target by acting on vimentin and inhibits metastasis [28].

The potential prognostic role of vimentin was described for TSCC and OSCC [29, 30]. In the first situation, vimentin among the EMT related proteins such as Snail, E- cadherin and N-cadherin are involved. In the second situation, an association between vimentin intense immunoexpression and a high risk for cervical lymph node metastatic potential was noticed. It was showed that vimentin-SOX 2 interrelation may represent an unfavorable risk factor for survival of head and neck squamous cell carcinoma. The loss of SOX2 expression induces cell motility by vimentin up-regulation [31].

Podoplanin, a 38 KDa type I transmembrane glycoprotein is overexpressed in different human cancers, including HNSCC.

An interrelation between histological grade differentiation and podoplanin immunoexpression was described in HNSCC. The main pattern of immunoexpression was in the cytoplasm and membrane with focal (mainly in the well differentiated OSCC) and diffuse distribution type (mainly in the moderately and poorly differentiated OSCC). The podoplanin was not expressed in the some of the well and poorly differentiated oral SCC cases. In all the moderately differentiated cases of SCC a positive reaction for podoplanin was noticed. The highest values for podoplanin with cytoplasm and membrane pattern expression was associated with poorly differentiated of oral SCC type. High levels of podoplanin expression was associated with high frequency of lymph node metastasis in OSCC [32]. A tendency of increasing podoplanin expression with decreasing of differentiation grade was noticed [33]. In OSCC was demonstrated the podoplanin involvement in the cytoskeleton remodeling, ECM degradation and tumor invasion. These are realized by co-location, co-ordination of podoplanin, Cdc42 and MT1-MMP in the invadopodia [34].

SCCs of the larynx and hypopharynx with high values of podoplanin expression were associated with an unfavorable prognosis also [35]. Podoplanin may have a predictive value of aggressiveness in HNSCC evolution, together with other markers such as EGFR and E-cadherin.

Another pathway through which podoplanin induces a decrease in overall survival was shown in the murine experimental models. Podoplanin expression in the OSCC tumors increased platelet activation and promotes intravascular platelet aggregation and intratumor platelet infiltration. The coagulation state is favorized [36].

4. Proliferation markers: p53 and Bcl2

P53 is a transcription factor that regulates the cell cycle, DNA repair and apoptosis. One of its main role is to maintain cellular integrity after DNA damage. Consecutive to this moment, p53 is regulated in a MDM2-dependent manner and activated by cell cycle checkpoint kinases type 1 and 2 [37]. In normal conditions, p53 may be expressed with a nuclear pattern in basal cells of the epithelium. In HNSCC p53 immunoexpression was described in 50% of the evaluated cases or more. Controversial data concerning p53/EGFR co-expression exists. In our data, 44% of larynx and 70.5% of pharynx cases co-expressed p53/ EGFR. All of the p53 positive cases co-expressed EGFR. These features were noticed by using a double immunohistochemical staining p 53/ EGFR. For larynx localization, p53/ EGFR co-expression was noticed mainly at the periphery of the tumor area (in all of the moderately differentiate cases- **Figure 1**, in 25% of well differentiate cases with much more reduced number of co-expressing cells, in 50% of poorly differentiated type). In corresponding lymph nodes of laryngeal tumors, the co-expressing cells were present in the immediate vicinity of the lymphoid tissue and to the periphery of tumor areas. In the center of tumor areas EGFR or p53 positive cells only were found, not co-expressing cells. The distribution pattern of the co-expressing cells from the hypopharynx may be noticed in the **Figure 2**. The distribution pattern of co-expressing cells to the periphery of tumor areas was found in the oropharynx, pharyngo-laryngeal and sinus nose localization. The co-expressing cells were absent in the naso-pharyngeal localization. A significant correlation was found between p53 intensity of expression and extranodal extension and tumor grade, mainly grades II and III [38, 39]. All of these p53/EGFR co-expression data may be useful for a better stratification of HNSCC, regarding the diagnostic but the therapy also.

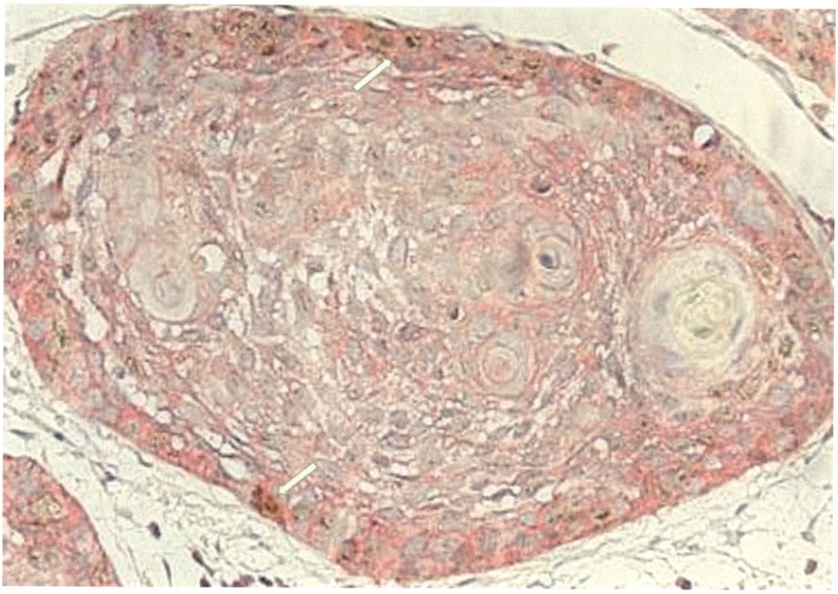

Figure 1.
p53/EGFR co- expression (white arrows) in tumor area in a case of moderately differentiated squamous cell carcinoma with larynx localization, double immunostaining p53/EGFR, ob.X40.

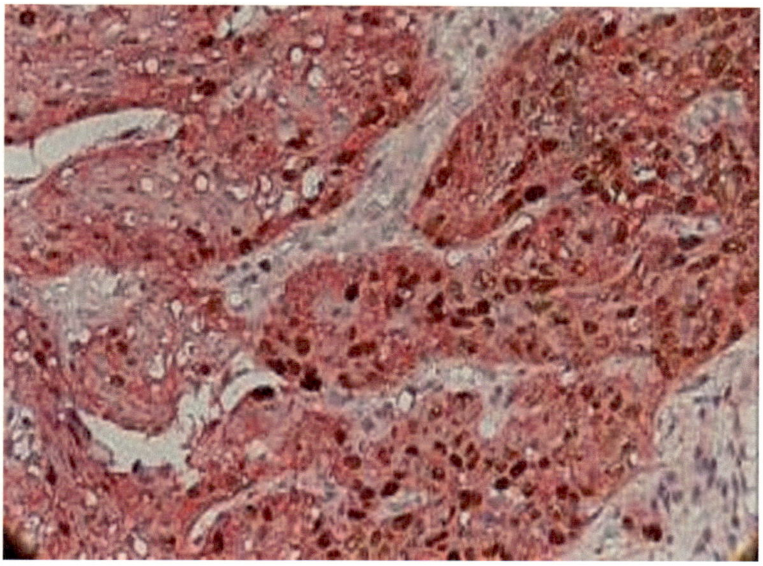

Figure 2.
EGFR/p53 immunoexpression, non-keratinized squamous cell carcinoma, moderately differentiated of hypopharynx, double immunostaining p53/EGFR, ob.X40.

The major pathways involved in the tumorigenesis of HNSCC include dysregulation of the following processes: cellular survival and proliferation, cell-cycle control, cellular differentiation and adhesion and invasion signaling. The main important factors involved in the cellular survival and proliferation are: TP53, HRAS, EGFR, PIK3CA. The functional inactivation of the p53 pathway was demonstrated in 80% of HNSCC, that why a therapeutic strategy which focus on the restoration of p53 function was developed for the HPV negative and HPV associated HNSCC. Unfortunately, the adenoviral p53 gene therapy has not been shown to be effective in clinical trials [40, 41].

Another important role of p 53 is the expression in the surgical margins. Pathology in the margin represent an considerable prognostic factor for relapse free survival (RFS) in the management of HNSCC treated with primary surgery. In the OSCC, a local recurrence value varies between 10 and 30% even if the histological status of margins is clear. The following surgical margins classification is used by surgeons and pathologists: involved margins (margin ≤1 mm), close margins (margin 1–5 mm) and clear margins (margin >5 mm) [42]. Severe dysplasia and invasive carcinoma needing additional resection while moderate and mild dysplasia do not. Evaluation of the p53 overexpression in histological resection margins of oral and oropharyngeal SCC demonstrated a 5.333 times higher chance of local recurrences if at least one margin overexpressed p53. P53 as an independent risk factor has been demonstrated in early OSCC with dysplastic surgical margin. It may be a useful marker for postoperative decision for these patients [43, 44].

Bcl-2 (B-cell lymphoma 2) encoded in humans by the Bcl2 gene is a member of the family of regulatory proteins that influence apoptosis through both pro and anti-apoptotic or inhibitory effects. Pro-survival Bcl-2 proteins (Bcl-2, Bcl-xL, MCL-1) inhibit Bcl-2 pro-apoptotic effectors (BAX and BAK).

The immunohistochemical evaluation of cases from our studies, revealed a relatively reduce number of bcl2 cases. The value of positive cases was close to 30%. The differences were noticed between anatomic areas. At the larynx, oropharynx, hypopharynx, nasopharynx, bcl 2expression in some of the cases was found. At the pharingo-larynx, nasal sinus, bcl2 expression was absent. Cases of well and poorly differentiated keratinized squamous cell carcinoma of the larynx were characterized by the absence of Bcl2 immunohistochemical expression in tumor cells. A similar appearance was noticed in the tumor cells of the corresponding lymph node. The Bcl2 immunoexpression had a score value 2 (10–30% positive tumor cells) in primary tumor and corresponding lymph node of the squamous keratinized moderately differentiated larynx carcinoma. The same value was found in the oropharynx. In the lymph node of the non-keratinized moderately differentiated type of the larynx squamous cell carcinoma more than 50% of bcl 2 positive tumor cells were noticed (a value 3 of the score).

In the hypopharynx localization isolated Bcl 2 positive tumor cells were found in the tumor areas (score value 1, with less than 10% Bcl2 positive tumor cells- **Figure 3**). An intense Bcl2 expression as intensity and value of the score was expressed in the stromal cells in the vicinity of tumor areas.

The highest value score of Bcl2 (value 3: more than 50% Bcl2 positive tumor cells- **Figure 4**) was present in the non-keratinized moderately differentiated squamous cell carcinoma with rhino-pharynx localization. In the group of EGFR positive cases, 3 sub groups were described: EGFR+/p53−/bcl2-, EGFR+/p53+/bcl2+ and EGFR+/p53+/bcl2−/with a significant correlation between N parameter and EGFR expression in this last subgroup. In the K5+/EGFR + cases significant correlation between bcl2 and M ($p = 0.01$) and N ($p = 0.04$) parameters were found. Other HNSCC immunohistochemistry data indicated a higher Bcl 2 expression, compare with our data, around 88% of evaluated cases. A significant correlation was reported between the Bcl2 expression and histological grade, lymph node involvement but not clinical stage. They noticed a significant association between p53+/Bcl2 + and histological grade, lymph node involvement [13, 45].

Other authors considered that immunohistochemical staining of Bcl2 is not significantly correlated with tumoral aggressiveness and prognosis to the patients diagnosed with laryngeal squamous cell carcinoma and treated with primary surgery [46]. The molecular mechanism and genetic basis of the development of larynx carcinoma have not been fully elucidated. Some data revealed the involvement of Bcl2-Hsp90beta in the anti-apoptotic progression of larynx carcinoma.

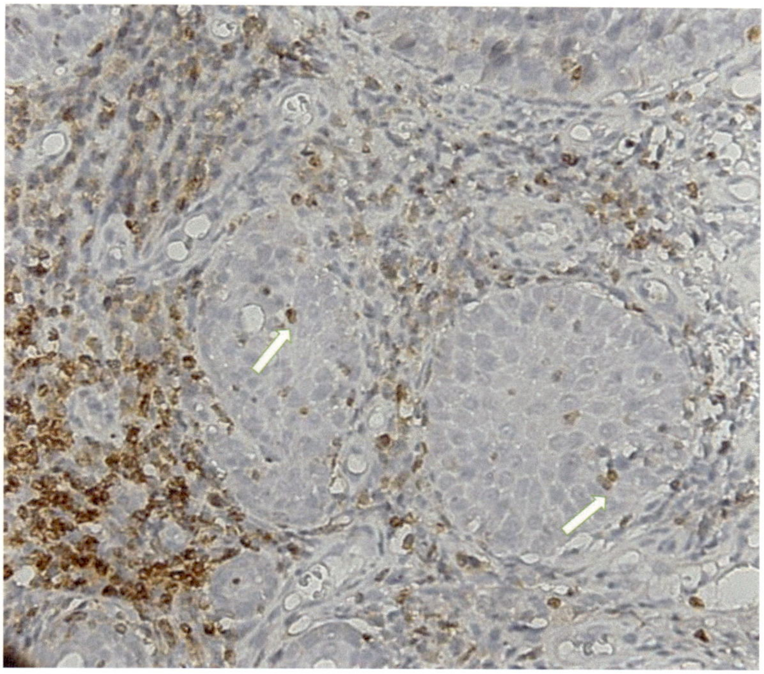

Figure 3.
Value 1 of Bcl2 immunoexpression score inside the tumor area (white arrows), in a moderately differentiated squamous cell carcinoma of the hypopharynx, Bcl2 immunostaining, ob.X40.

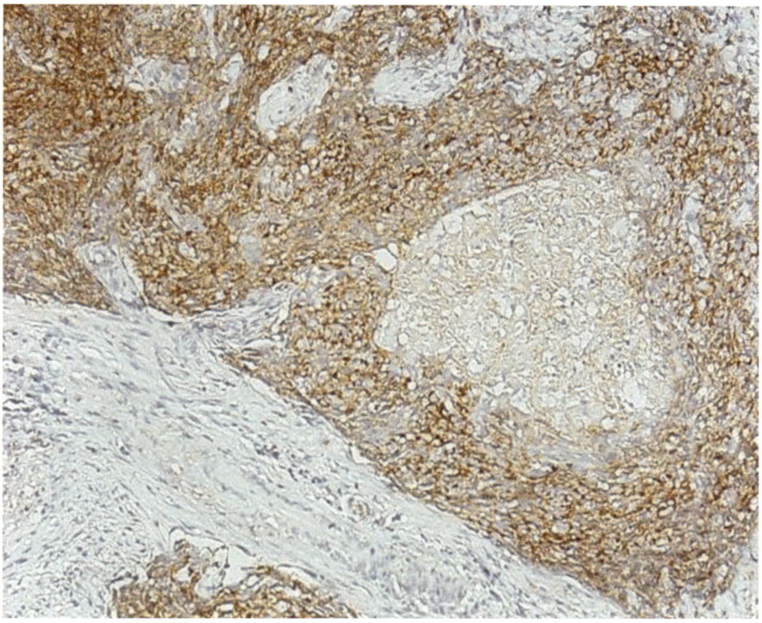

Figure 4.
Value 3 of Bcl-2 expression score in a moderately differentiated, non-keratinized squamous cell carcinoma of the rhinopharynx, Bcl2 immunostaining, ob. X 20.

The disruption of Bcl2-Hsp90beta interaction inhibited the anti-apoptotic ability of Bcl2 and reduced the capsize activation in larynx carcinomas [47].

It was demonstrated the role of miR-15a as a suppressor in HPV positive by targeting bcl2 in HSCC [48]. The effect of Navitoclax (a small inhibitor molecule of Bcl-2/Bcl-xL), in high doses was the death of HNSCC cells. But a limited effect was found in combination with radiation or cisplatin. Co-inhibition of MCL-1 was required to improve approaches targeting Bcl-2/Bcl-xL in HNSCC [49].

By evaluate two groups of metastatic and non-metastatic primary OSCC, Pavithra et al. [50] found no significant difference in the expression of Bcl2 between the two groups. They sustained that evaluation of Bcl2 along with other apoptotic proteins could define the role in prognosis and pathogenesis of OSCC.

Taking into account all these data, bcl2 alone or together with p53 expression may still represent some important markers for tumor agressivity and survival rates in the conditions of a better stratification of the patients.

5. Growth factors and their receptors

Some of the most important growth factors already described to be involved in the prognosis or therapy resistance of HNSCC are: epidermal growth factor (EGF) and it receptor EGFR, vascular endotelial growth factor (VEGF) and VEGFR 1 and 2 mainly, platelet derived growth factor (PDGF AA) and PDGFR alpha, nerve growth factor (NGF) and transforming growth factor beta (TGF-beta).

There are some molecular-targeted therapies used in the treatment of head and neck squamous cell carcinoma. The molecular targeted therapy such as Cetuximab, panitumumab, zalutumumab and nimotuzumab acts on EGFR monoclonal antibodies; Gefitinib, erlotinib, lapatinib, afatinib, dacomitinib inhibit EGFR tirosin kinase receptors; Bevacizumab (VEGF inhibitor); Sorafenib, sunitinib, vandetanib (VEGFR inhibitors); Rapamycin, temsirolimus, everolimus, torin 1, PP242 and PP30 (PI3K/AKT/mTOR pathway); Pembrolizumab and nivolumab (anti-PD-1).

The EGFR ligands such as EGF, transforming growth factor alpha (TGFA), heparin-binding EGF-like growth factor (HBEGF), amphiregulin (AREG), betacellulin (BTC), epiregulin (EREG) and epigen (EPGN) are involved in tumor growth, invasion and metastatic process through EGFR activation. In HNSCC, these ligands/receptors are deregulated. It was noticed an important correlation between mRNA levels of four EGFR ligands and the poor prognosis in HNSCC. The inhibiting EGF- induced AREG expression was proposed as a new treatment option in HNSCC [51].

The EGFR targeting monoclonal antibody, Cetuximab was FDA approved for HNSCC treatment in 2006. But, despite the advances in therapy, the overall five years survival rate of patients with advanced HNSCC remains relatively reduced, around 40–50%. Some data described mutations in various oncogenes and tumor suppressor genes in HNSCC profile, as following: PIK3CA (21%), HRAS (4%), TP53 (72%), CDKN (22%), FBXW7 (5%), KMT2D (MLL2) (18%) and PTEN (2%). PI3K/AKT pathway responsible of proliferation, survive and cell differentiation exhibit alterations in around 34% of patients diagnosed with HNSCC. This pathway may be responsible for tumor escape during EGFR targeting in HNSCC. It was demonstrated the role of PIK3CA and RAS mutations in predicted cetuximab resistance in the first line recurrent and/or metastatic setting and the role of PTEN protein expression loss in predicted resistance to cetuximab when combined to radiotherapy [52].

VEGF- A and the others family members (VEGF-B, VEGF-C, VEGF-D) are overexpressed in the majority of HNSCC cases. They act by inducing tumor growth by changing the microvascular density, favorizing cell migration and metastasis. The reduced sensitivity to radiation and progression of HNSCC is associated with stimulation of angiogenesis by tumor cells that undergo radiotherapy. The results of phase I and II clinical trials of Bevacizumab and erlotinib combined administration indicated an increase of median survival by seven months. One of the therapeutic agents, which induce autophagy and inhibits tumor growth was Sorafenib, a serine-threonine protein kinase inhibitor b-Raf, C-Raf, VEGF and PDGFR. Sunitinib, a small molecule kinase inhibitor of VEGFR, PDGFR and c-kit tyrosine kinase has a reduced effect if it is use as monotherapy but associated with Cetuximab favorized the decrease of tumor cell proliferation and an increase of cell differentiation. Vandetanib, which targeted on EGFR, VEGFR2, RTK used in combination with cisplatin and radiotherapy reduced the resistance to EGFR inhibitors in preclinical trials [53]. It was demonstrated also the role of the preoperative or postoperative serum levels of VEGF as a predictive factor for recurrence, disease- free and overall survival of patients with HNSCC [54]. The results obtained on culture cells support the application in clinical practice of the levels of the VEGFR promoters. Methylation of VEGFR1 and VEGFR3 promoters correlated with poor prognosis. It was established a link between methylation of the VEGFR2 promoter and lymph node metastasis [55].

Concerning PDGF and their receptor it was found a prognostic role of PDGF serum level in patients with OSCC and a worse prognostic of HNSCC patients induced by the presence of PDGFR-alfa expression in the tumor microenvironment [56, 57].

Both normal and malignant epithelial cells expressed NGF receptors and NGF gene. Neurotrophins are involved in perineural growth in HNSCC, a pathway of tumor progression associated with poor prognosis. Neurotrophins link to low affinity nerve growth factor (LNGFR/p75 neurotrophin receptor-p75 NTR) or to the high affinity Trk (tropomyosin related kinase) tyrosine kinase receptors. P75 NTR was described in an undifferentiated cell population of oral leukoplakia and in OSCC where was associate with a poor prognosis. P75NTR contribute to drug resistance, by involvement in multiple signaling pathways. A correlation between neurotrophin receptor tyrosine kinase (NTRK2) overexpression and epithelial to mesenchymal transition in HNSCC tumor cells was found. It seems that p75NTR might related with NGF -independent therapy resistance in HNSCC, while NTRK1 might transduce a survival signal on NGF and improved cell survival after cell cycle arrest [58].

Another important growth factor with increased importance in HNSCC is hepatocyte growth factor (HGF) and its receptor c-MET. The overexpression of HGF was commonly reported in HNSCC cases. C-MET was overexpressed in lymph node metastasis of HNSCC. C-MET encodes mesenchymal epithelial transition factor which favorized invasion and metastatic potential in cancers. Their overexpression may be associated with worse prognostic and reduced overall survival rate. EGFR and c-MET share common downstream pathways: RAS-RAF-MAPK and PI3K-AKT-mTOR. In the patients with resistance to EGFR targeted therapies c-MET/HGF inhibitors may represent an alternative solution. Capmatinib as monotherapy and Ficlatuzumab combined with Cetuximab are some of c-MET/HGF axis therapeutic solutions.

Transforming growth factor beta realized homeostasis between the proliferation and apoptosis of normal epithelial cell by Smads or Smad independent downstream pathways. Tumor suppression and tumor promotion is the main role of TGF beta in HNSCC [59].

6. The afferent stroma proliferation. The mast cell, blood vessels and lymphatic vessels involvement

The stromal component of the tumor microenvironment contains different cells types such as: cancer associated fibroblast, macrophages, regulatory T cells and mast cells.

Regulatory T cells recruitment is regulated by chemokines and associated receptors (CCL28-CCR10 and CXCL12-CXCR4). The immunohistochemical specific markers of these cells are CD4 and CD25. It was identified a subgroup of Tregs, TIM3, with high levels of T-cell immunoglobulin and mucin domain-3. It was notice that these cells are linked with resistance to radiotherapy and their number decrease after PD-1 monoclonal antibody administration. In HNSCC, a high number of Tregs induces a negative prognostic [60].

Described for the first time by Ehrlich in 1878, mast cells differ through their localization and content, depending on their phenotype: connective tissue MCs and mucosal MCs. Mast cells granules contained preformed mediators such as: tryptase, chymase, cathepsin G, histamine, heparin, serotonin, IL-16, and TNF alpha. Mediators synthesized after mast cell activation are interleukines (IL1, IL 3, IL4, IL 5, IL6, IL 8, IL 10, IL 13, IL 16, platelet activating factor, RANTES, MIF 1 alpha) and arachidonic acid metabolites, prostaglandin and leukotriene C4 [61, 62].

In HNSCC, some authors noticed a decrease in mast cell number associated with advanced histological grade in OSCC, other found a significant correlation between mast cells density and G1, G2 histological grade in larynx carcinoma [63, 64].

By the content of their granules such as VEGF or other substances with angiogenic properties, mast cells may stimulate angiogenesis. In the larynx carcinoma, the differentiation grade was correlated with mast cell density but not with the microvascular density [64]. Other data indicated a higher MVD in HNSCC compare with MVD values noticed in dysplasia of the upper respiratory tract epithelium. No significant correlation was found between MVD/CD34 values and local invasiveness (the T feature) in HNSCC [65]. Increased values of MVD and mast cell density were present in OSCC compare with leukoplakia with and without dysplasia [66].

Lymphangiogenesis is the process of new lymphatic vessel formation. The growth factors such as VEGF-C, VEGF -D, PDGF-BB and HGF may influence the formation of new lymphatic vessels. Both lymphatic and microvascular density in peritumoral area may have a prognostic value. Some data demonstrated that peritumoral MVD was associated with metastasis and LMVD was inversely related to both metastasis and progression in HNSCC [67]. Other authors compared the intra and peritumoral lymphatic microvascular density and found a significantly lower density in the peri-tumoral areas. They found significant correlation between LMVD values (intra and peri-tumoral) and differentiation degree. From clinical parameters, an important correlation between total LMVD and lymph node status, but not tumor stage was reported [68]. These observations were reconfirmed by other study which reported an important correlation between both high intra-tumoral and peritumoral LVD and lymph node metastasis. The morphology of peri-tumoral lymphatic vessels was similar, with a large lumen, like in the previously study, but the number of lymphatic vessels was higher in peritumoral area compared with intra-tumoral area, opposite to previous study [69].

These results support the importance of the lymphangiogenesis and lymphatic vascular density as risk and prognostic factors of the patients with lymph node metastasis.

7. Conclusions

From the mentioned data results the necessity of a better stratification of HNSCC. The novel molecular techniques of the surgical margins can offer a more accurate risk assessment. The results of genetic and molecular biology studies may outline the criteria for the targeted therapy as a fundamental method of cancer treatment in the future.

Conflict of interest

The authors declare no conflict of interest.

Author details

Amalia Raluca Ceausu[1*], Eugen Radu Boia[2], Eugen Sorin Boia[3],
Anca Maria Cimpean[1] and Marius Raica[1]

1 Department of Microscopic Morphology/Histology, Angiogenesis Research Center, "Victor Babes" University of Medicine and Pharmacy, Timisoara, Romania

2 ENT Department, "Victor Babes" University of Medicine and Pharmacy Timişoara, Timisoara, Romania

3 Department of Pediatric Surgery and Ortopedics, "Victor Babeş" University of Medicine and Pharmacy Timişoara, Timisoara, Romania

*Address all correspondence to: ra.ceausu@umft.ro

References

[1] Bray F, Ferlay J, Soerjomataram I, Siegel RL, Torre LA, Jemal A. Global cancer statistics 2018: GLOBOCAN estimates of incidence and mortality worldwide for 36 cancers in 185 countries. CA Cancer J. Clin. 2018; 68: 394-424. DOI: 10.3322/caac.21492

[2] Leemans CR, Snijders PJF, Brakenhoff RH. The molecular landscape of head and neck cancer. Nat. Rev. Cancer. 2018; 18: 269-282. DOI: 10.138/nrc.2018.11

[3] Tolstong G, Simon C. Trends in surgical research in head and neck cancer. Curr. Treat. Options Oncol. 2017; 18: 38-51. DOI: 10.1007/s11864-017-0475-z

[4] Chung CH, Parker JS, Karaca G, Wu J, Funkhouser WK, Moore D, Butterfoss D, Xiang D, Zanation A, Yin X, Shockley WW, Weissler MC, Dressler LG, Shores CG, Yarbrough WG, Perou CM. Molecular classification of head and neck squamous cell carcinomas using patterns of gene expression. Cancer Cell. 2004; 5: 489-500. DOI: 10.1016/S1535-6108 (04) 00112-6

[5] Walter V, Yin X, Wilkerson MD, Cabanski CR, Zhao N, Du Y, Ang MK, Hayward MC, Salazar AH, Hoadley KA, Fritchie K, Sailey CJ, Weissler MC, Shockley WW, Zanation AM, Hackman T, Thorne LB, Funkhouser WD, Muldrew KL, Olshan AF, Randell SH, Wright FA, Shores CG, Hayes DN. Molecular subtypes in head and neck cancer exhibit distinct patterns of chromosomal gain and loss of canonical cancer genes. Plos One. 2013; 8(2): e56823. DOI:10.1371/journal.pone.0056823

[6] Keck MK, Zuo Z, Khattri A, Stricker TP, Brown CD, Imanguli M, Rieke D, Endhardt K, Fang P, Bragelmann J, DeBoer R, El-Dinali M, Aktolga S, Lei Z, Tan P, Rozen SG, Salgia R, Weichselbaum RR, Lingen MW, Story MD, Ang KK, Cohen EEW, White PK, Vokes EE, Seiwert TY. Integrative analysis of head and neck cancer identifies two biologically distinct HPV and three non-HPV subtypes. Clin. Cancer Res. 2015; 21: 870-881. DOI: 10.1158/1078-0432.CCR-14-2481

[7] De Cecco L, Nicolau M, Giannoccaro M, Daidone MG, Bossi P, Locati L, Licitra L, Canevari S. Head, and neck cancer subtypes with biological and clinical relevance: meta-analysis of gene- expression data. Oncotarget. 2015; 6: 9627-9642.DOI: 10.18632/oncotarget.3301

[8] Canning M, Guo G, Yu M, Myint C, Groves MW, Byrd JK, Cui Y. Heterogeneity of the head and neck squamous cell carcinoma immune landscape and its impact on immunotherapy. Front Cell Dev Biol. 2019; 7:52. DOI: 10.3389/fcell.2019.00052

[9] Brierley JD, Gospodarowicz MK, Wittekind C. TNM Classification of malignant tumors. 8th ed. UICC: Wiley; 2017. 272 p.

[10] Westra WH, Lewis JS. Update from the 4th edition of the World Health Organization classification of head and neck tumours: Oropharynx. Head Neck Pathol. 2017; 11 (1): 41-47. DOI: 10.1007/s12105-017-0793-2

[11] Barnes L, Eveson JW, Reichart P, Sidransky D. World Health Organization Classification of Tumours. 9th ed. WHO: IARC Press; 2005. 422 p.

[12] Thompson L. Head and neck pathology. Foundatios in Diagnostic Pathology Series: Churchill Livingstone, Elsevier, 2006. 640 p.

[13] Cimpean AM, Balica AR, Doros CI, Balica NC, Gaje PN, Popovici AR, Raica M. Epidermal growth factor receptor (EGFR) and keratin 5 (K5): versatile keyplayers defining prognostic and therapeutic sub-classes of head and neck squamous cell carcinomas. Cancer Genomics and Proteomics. 2016; 13 (1): 75-81

[14] Boia S, Boia ER, Ceausu AR, Balica NC, Mederle OA. HPV 18 associated E-cadherin expression in head and neck squamous cell carcinoma. Rev Chim. 2018; 69 (10): 2638-2641. DOI: 10.37358/RC.18.10.6596

[15] El-Naggar AK, Chan J, Grandis J, Takata T, Slootweg P. WHO classification of head and neck tumours. 4th ed. WHO: IARC Press; 2017. 400 p.

[16] Broglie MA, Dulguerov P, Henke G, Siano M, Putora PM, Simon C, Zwahlen D, Huber GF, Ballerini G, Beffa L, Giger R, Rothschild S, Negri SV, Elicin O. A review of controversial issues in the management of head and neck cancer: a Swiss multidisciplinary and multi-institutional patterns of care study -part 4 (biomarkers). Front Oncol. 2019; 9:1128-1133. DOI: 10.3389/fonc.2019.01128

[17] Grimm M. Prognostic value of clinicopathological parameters and outcome in 484 patients with oral squamous cell carcinoma: microvascular invasion (V+) is an independent prognostic factor for OSCC. Clin Transl Oncol. 2012; 14: 870-880. DOI: 10.1007/s12094-012-0867-2

[18] Coelho BA, Peterle GT, Santos M, Agostini LP, Maia LL, Stur E, Silva CVM, Mendes SO, Almanca CCJ, Freitas FV, Borcoi AR, Archanjo AB, Mercante AMC, Nunes FD, Carvalho MB, Tajara EH, Louro ID, Conforti-Silva AMA. Keratins 17 and 19 expression as prognostic markers in oral squamous cell carcinoma. Genet Mol Res. 2015; 14(4): 15123-15132. DOI: 10.4238/2015.November.24.21

[19] Tang KD, Kenny L, Perry C, Frazer I, Punyadeera C. The overexpression of salivary cytokeratins as potential diagnostic biomarkers in head and neck squamous cell carcinomas. Oncotarget. 2017; 8(42): 72272-72280. DOI: 10.18632/oncotarget.19731

[20] Dahiya K, Dhankhar R. Updated overview of current biomarkers in head and neck carcinoma. World J Methodol. 2016; 6: 77-86. DOI: 10.5662/wjm.v6.i1.77

[21] Vasca V, Vasca E, Freiman P, Marian D, Luce A, Mesolella M, Caraglia M, Ricciardiello F, Duminica T. Keratin 5 expression in squamocellular carcinoma of the head and neck. Oncol. Lett. 2014; 8 (6): 2501-2504. DOI: 10.3892/ol.2014.2591

[22] Savagner P. The epithelial-mesenchymal transition (EMT) phenomenon. Annals of Oncology. 2010; 21 (7): 89-92. DOI: 10.1093/annonc/mdq292

[23] Gaiser MR, Hirsch D, Gaiser T. Loss of epithelial cell adhesion molecule (EpCAM) in infiltrative basal cell carcinoma. Int J Clin Exp. Pathol. 2018; 11 (1): 406-412. Published 2018 Jan 1.

[24] Sequeira I, Neves JF, Carrero D, Peng Q, Palasz N, Liakath-Ali K, Lord GM, Morgan PR, Lombardi G, Watt FM. Immunomodulatory role of keratin 76 in oral and gastric cancer. Nat. Commun. 2018; 9: 3437. DOI: 10.1038/s41467-018-05872

[25] Srivastava SS, Alam H, Patil SJ, Shrinivasan R, Raikundalia S, Chaudhari PR, Vaidya MM. Keratin 5/14 mediated cell differentiation and transformation are regulated by TAp63 and Notch-1 in oral squamous cell carcinoma-derived cells. Oncol

Rep 2018; 39: 2393-2401. DOI: 10.3892/or.2018.6298

[26] Litvinov SV, Balzar M, Winter MJ, Bakker HA, Briaire-de Bruijn IH, Prins F, Fleuren GJ, Warnaar SO. Epithelial cell adhesion molecule (Ep-CAM) modulates cell-cell interactions mediated by classic cadherins. J Cell Biol. 1997; 139: 1337-1348. DOI: 10.1083/jcb. 139.5.1337

[27] Chaw SY, Majeed AJ, Chan A, Stein S, Farah CS. Epithelial to mesenchymal transition (EMT) biomarkers- E-cadherin, beta-catenin, APC, and vimentin – in oral squamous cell carcinogenesis and transformation. Oral Oncol. 2012 ; 48 (10) : 997-1006. DOI : 10.1016/j.oraloncology.2012.05.011

[28] Dong Y, Zheng Y, Wang C, Ding X, Du Y, Liu L, Zhang W, Zhong Y, Wu Y, Song X. MiR-876-5p modulates head and neck squamous cell carcinoma metastasis and invasion by targeting vimentin. Cancer Cell Int. 2018; 18: 121. DOI: 10.1186/s12935-018-0619-7

[29] Liu PF, Kang BH, Wu YM, Sun JH, Yen LM, Fu TY, Lin YC, Liou HH, Lin YS, Sie HC, Hsieh IC, Tseng YK, Shu CW, Hsieh DY, Ger LP. Vimentin is a potential prognostic factor for tongue squamous cell carcinoma among five epithelial-mesenchymal transition related proteins. Plos One. 2017; 12(6): e0178581. DOI: 10.1371/ journal. pone. 0178581

[30] Liu S, Liu L, Ye W, Ye D, Wang T, Guo W, Liao Y, Xu D, Song H, Zhang L, Zhu H, Deng J, Zhang Z. High vimentin expression associated with lymph node metastasis and predicated a poor prognosis in oral squamous cell carcinoma. Sci Rep. 2016; 6: 38834. DOI: 10.1038/srep38834

[31] Bayo A, Jou A, Stenzinger A, Shao C, Gross M, Jensen A, Grabe N, Mende CH, Rados PV, Debus J, Weichert W, Plinkert PK, Lichter P, Freier K, Hess J. Loss of SOX2 expression induces cell motility via vimentin up-regulation and is an unfavorable risk factor for survival of head and neck squamous cell carcinoma. Mol Oncol. 2015; 9(8): 1704-1719. DOI: 10.1016/j.molonc.2015.05.006

[32] Prasad B, Kashyap B, Babu GS, Kumar GR, Manyam R. Expression of podoplanin in different grades of oral squamous cell carcinoma. Ann Med Health Sci Res. 2015; 5(4): 299-304. DOI: 10.4103/2141-9248.160181

[33] Deepa AG, Bindu JN, Varun BR. Podoplanin expression in oral potentially malignant disorders and oral squamous cell carcinoma. Journal of Clinical and Experimental Dentistry. 2017; 9(12): e 1418-e 1424. DOI: 10.4317/jced.54213

[34] Li YY, Zhou CX, Gao Y. Podoplanin promotes the invasion of oral squamous cell carcinoma in coordination with MT1-MMP and Rho GTPases. Am J Cancer Res. 2015; 5(2): 514-529

[35] Voelker HU, Hintermer I, Strehl A, Scheich M. Prognostic potential of the expression of podoplanin (D2-40) within cells of squamous cell carcinoma of the larynx and hypopharynx. World J Oncol. 2020; 11(2): 65-71. DOI: 10.14740/wjon1259

[36] Lee NY, Yu NY, Lee SH, Tsai HJ, Wu CC, Cheng JC, Chen PD, Wang RY, Tseng CP. Podoplanin promotes cancer -associated thrombosis and contributes to unfavorable overall survival in an ectopic xenograft mouse model of oral cancer. Biomed J. 2020; 43(2): 146-162. DOI: 10.1016/j.bj.2019.07.001

[37] Wu D, Prives C. Relevance of the p53-MDM 2 axis to aging. Cell Death Differ. 2018; 25:169-179. DOI: 1038/cdd.2017.187

[38] Hashmi AA, Hussain ZF, Hashmi SK, Irfan M, Khan EY,

Faridi N, Khan A, Edhi MM. Immunohistochemical over expression of p53 in head and neck squamous cell carcinoma: clinical and prognostic significance. BMC Res Notes 2018; 11: 433. DOI: 10.1186/s13104-018-3547-7

[39] Boia ER. Clinical-pathological and historical features of latero-cervical lymphadenopathy [thesis]. Marioara Poenaru: Victor Babes University of Medicine and Pharmacy; 2014.

[40] Castellanos MR, Pan Q. Novel p53 therapies for head and neck cancer. World J Otorhinolaryngol Head Neck Surg. 2016; 2(2): 68-75. DOI: 10.1016/j.wjorl.2016.05.005

[41] Zhou G, Liu Z, Myers JN. TP53 mutations in head and neck squamous cell carcinoma and their impact on disease progression and treatment response. J Cell Biochem. 2016; 117(12): 2682-2692. DOI: 10.1002/jcb.25592

[42] Prya SR, D'Cruz AK, Pai PS. Cut margins and disease control in oral cancers. J Cancer Res Ther. 2012; 8(1): 74-79. DOI: 10.4103/0973-1482.95178

[43] Yang XH, Ding L, Fu Y, Chen S, Zhang L, Zhang XX, Huang XF, Lu ZY, Ni YH, Hu QG. p53 positive expression in dysplastic surgical margins is a predictor of tumor recurrence in patients with early oral squamous cell carcinoma. Cancer Manag Res 2019; 11: 1465-1472. DOI: 10.2147/ CMAR.S192500

[44] Shah AK. Postoperative pathologic assessment of surgical margins in oral cancer: a contemporary review. J Oral Maxillofac Pathol. 2018; 22(1): 78-85. DOI: 10.4103/jomfp. JOMFP_185_16

[45] Taneja K, Gupta S, Chauhan AK, Kalra R, Arora A, Arora S, Sen R. Expression of p53 and bcl2 in squamous cell carcinoma of head and neck. Archives of Clinical and Experimental Surgery. 2016; 5: 160-168. DOI: 10.5455/aces.20151006071751

[46] Gioacchini FM, Ciufelli MA, Rubini C, Magliulo G, Re M. Prognostic value of Bcl2 expression in squamous cell carcinoma of the larynx: a systematic review. The International Journal of Biological Markers. 2018; 30: 155-160. DOI: 10.5301/jbm.5000116

[47] Li S, Li J, Hu T, Zhang C, Lv X, He S, Yan H, Tan Y, Wen M, Lei M, Zuo J. Bcl2 overexpression contributes to laryngeal carcinoma cell survival by forming a complex with Hsp90beta. Oncology Reports. 2016; 37: 849-856. DOI: 10.3892/or.2016.5295

[48] Lu W, Feng L, Zhang Y, Ma Y, Li P, Wang Y, Du Y, Chen X, Wu S, Zhao G, Lou W. miR-15a induces cell apoptosis by targeting Bcl2L2 and Bcl2 in HPV positive hypopharyngeal squamous cell carcinoma. Oncol. Rep. 2016; 36(4): 2169-2176. DOI: 10.3892/or.2016.5049

[49] Ow TJ, Fulcher CD, Thomas C, Broin PO, Lopez A, Reyna DE, Smith RV, Sarta C, Prystowsky MB, Schlecht NF, Schiff BA, Rosenblatt G, Belbin TJ, Harris TM, Childs GC, Kawachi N, Guha C, Gavathiotis E. Optimal targeting of Bcl-family proteins in head and neck squamous cell carcinoma requires inhibition of both Bcl-xL and MCL-1. Oncotarget. 2019; 10: 494-510. DOI: 10.18632/oncotarget.26563

[50] Pavithra V, Kumari K, Haragannavar VC, Rao RS, Nambiar S, Augustine D, Sowmya SV. Possible role of Bcl2 expression in metastatic and non -metastatic oral squamous cell carcinoma. J Clin Diagn Res. 2017; 11(9): 51-54. DOI: 10.7860/JCDR/2017/29363.10601

[51] Gao J, Ulekleiv CH, Halstensen TS. Epidermal growth factor (EGF) receptor ligand based molecular staging predicts prognosis in head and neck squamous cell carcinoma partly due to deregulated

EGF- induced amphiregulin expression. Journal of Experimental &Clinical Cancer Research. 2016; 35:151. DOI: 10.1186/s13046-016-0422-z

[52] Leblanc O, Vacher S, Lecerf C, Jeannot E, Klijanienko J, Berger F, Hoffmann C, Calugaru V, Badois N, Chilles A, Lesnik M, Krhili S, Bieche I, Le Tourneau C, Kamal M. Biomarkers of cetuximab resistance in patients with head and neck squamous cell carcinoma. Cancer Biol Med. 2020; 17(1): 208-217. DOI: 10.20892/j.issn.2095-3941.2019.0153

[53] Kozakiewicz P, Szatkowska LG. Application of molecular targeted therapies in the treatment of head and neck squamous cell carcinoma. Oncology Letters. 2018; 15(5): 7497-7505. DOI: 10.3892/ol.2018.8300

[54] Khademi B, Soleimanpour M, Ghaderi A, Mohammadianpanah M. Prognotic and predictive value of serum vascular endothelial growth factor (VEGF) in squamous cell carcinoma of the head and neck. Oral Maxillofac Surg. 2014; 18(2): 187-196. DOI: 10.1007/s10006-013-0402-9

[55] Misawa Y, Misawa K, Kawasaki H, Imai A, Mochizuki D, Ishikawa R, Endo S, Mima M, Kanazawa T, Iwashita T, Mineta H. Evaluation of epigenetic inactivation of vascular endothelial growth factor receptors in head and neck squamous cell carcinoma. Tumor Biology. 2017; 7:1-10. DOI: 10.1177/1010428317711657

[56] Lin LH, Lin JS, Yang CC, Cheng HW, Chang KW, Liu CJ. Overexpression of platelet-derived growth factor and its receptor are correlated with oral tumorigenesis and poor prognosis in oral squamous cell carcinoma. Int J Mol Sci. 2020; 21(7): 2360. DOI: 10.3390/ijms21072360

[57] Watts TL, Cui R, Szaniszlo P, Resto AV, Powell DW, Pinchuk I, PDGF-AA mediates mesenchymal stromal cell chemotaxis to the head and neck squamous cell carcinoma tumor microenvironment. J Transl Med. 2016; 14: 337. DOI: 10.1186/s12967-016-1091-6

[58] Dudas J, Dietl W, Romani A, Reinold S, Glueckert R, Fischer AS, Deiaco D, Chacko LJ, Tuertscher R, Schartinger VH, Riechelmann H. Nerve growth factor (NGF) receptor survival axis in head and neck squamous cell carcinoma. Int J Mol Sci. 2018; 19(6): 1771. DOI : 10.3390/ijms19061771

[59] Pang X, Tang YL, Liang XH. Transforming growth factor- beta signaling in head and neck squamous cell carcinoma: insights into cellular responses. Oncol Lett. 2018; 16(4): 4799-4806. DOI: 10.3892/ol.2018.9319

[60] Wang HC, Chan LP, Cho SF. Targeting the immune microenviroment in the treatment of head and neck squamous cell carcinoma. Front Oncol. 2019; 9: 1084. DOI: 10.3389/fonc.2019.01084

[61] Gaje PN, Ceausu AR, Jitariu A, Stratul SI, Rusu LC, Popovici AR, Raica M. Mast cells: key players in the shadow in oral inflammation and in squamous cell carcinoma of the oral cavity. Bio Med Research International. 2016; DOI: 10.1155.2016/9235080

[62] Peltanova B, Raudenska M, Masarik M. Effect of tumor microenvironment on pathogenesis of the head and neck squamous cell carcinoma: a systematic review. Mol Cancer. 2010; 18: 63. DOI: 10.1186/s12943-019-0983-5

[63] Balica NC, Ceausu AR, Gaje PN, Doros C, Poenaru M. Microvessel and mast cell densities in malignant laryngeal neoplasm. Archives of Biological Sciences. 2014. 66(3): 1163-1169. DOI: 10.2298/ABS1403163B

[64] Belgaumi UI, Patil S, Baad R, Vibhute N, Kadashetti V, Sushma B,

Kamate W. A study of association of mast cell count in different grades of oral squamous cell carcinoma. Ann Med Health Sci Res. 2017; 7:102-105.

[65] Szafarowski T, Sierdzinski J, Szxzepanski MJ, Whiteside TL, Ludwing N, Krzeski A. Microvessel density in head and neck squamous cell carcinoma. Eur Arch Otorhinolaryngol. 2018; 275 (7): 1845-1851. DOI: 10.1007/s00405-018-4996-2

[66] Laishram D, Rao K, Devi HSU, Priya NS, Smitha T, Sheethal HS. Mast cells and angiogenesis in malignant and premalignant oral lesions: an immunohistochemical study. J Oral Maxxilofac Pathol. 2017; 21 (2): 229-238. DOI: 10.4103/jomfp.JOMFP_111_15

[67] Evans M, Baddour HM, Magliocca KR, Muller S, Nannapaneni S, Chen AY, Kim S, Chen Z, Shin DM, Wang AY, Saba NF, Chen ZG. Prognostic implications of peritumoral vasculature in head and neck cancer. Cancer Medicine. 2019; 8:147-154. DOI: 10.1002/cam4.1910

[68] Cirligeriu L, Cimpean AM, Raica M, Doros CI. Dual role of podoplanin in oral cancer development. In vivo. 2014; 28(3): 341-347

[69] Parmar P, Marwah N, Parshad S. Clinicopathological significance of tumor lymphatic vessel density in head and neck squamous cell carcinoma. Indian Journal of Otolaryngology and head and neck surgery: official publication of the Association of Otolaryngologists of India. 2018. 70(1): 102-110. DOI: 10.1007/s12070-017-1216-0

Chapter 2

Pediatric Head and Neck Malignancies

Dustin A. Silverman, Ross Wanner, Patrick Walz, Matthew O. Old and Kris R. Jatana

Abstract

Head and neck malignancies are a part of the differential diagnosis of head and neck masses seen in the pediatric age group. It is critical to make prompt diagnosis and employ proper treatment. We will review the most common malignant pathologies as well as their specific clinical presentations and management. Centers that are able to provide multidisciplinary care for pediatric patients with head and neck pathology can help achieve the best outcomes.

Keywords: pediatric tumor, malignancy, neck mass, pediatric cancer, head and neck cancer

1. Introduction

Head and neck malignancies are rare within the pediatric population and represent 12% of all pediatric cancers according to the National Cancer Institute's Surveillance, Epidemiology, and End Results (SEER) database [1]. While epithelial tumors are more common in adults, childhood tumors are more frequently derived from mesenchymal and endothelial cells. Genetic conditions, previous chemotherapy, or exposure to ionizing radiation predispose this population to both primary and secondary malignancies, but the cumulative environmental carcinogen exposures (e.g. cigarette smoke inhalation, ultraviolet radiation) are much less common given the patients' younger ages [2].

The most common pediatric head and neck cancers include lymphoma (Hodgkin and non-Hodgkin), rhabdomyosarcoma, thyroid carcinoma, nasopharyngeal carcinoma, and salivary gland malignancies (**Figure 1**). While other malignancies such as neuroblastoma, neuroendocrine tumors, various soft-tissue sarcomas, cutaneous tumors, and metastases infrequently manifest within the head and neck region, a complete and thorough discussion of these cancers is outside the scope of this review and are covered elsewhere throughout literature. The primary aim of this review is to highlight the more common head and neck childhood malignancies and present a focused examination of the etiology, presentation, workup, and treatment of these conditions.

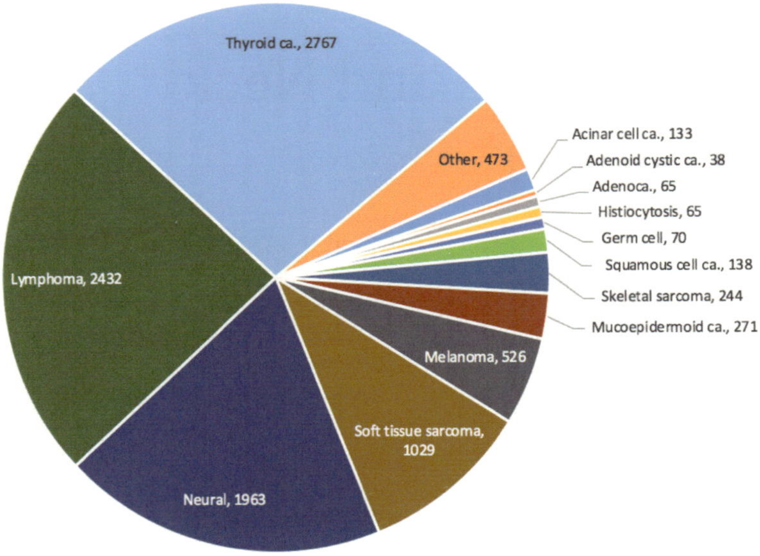

Figure 1.
Childhood head and neck malignancies by incidence 1973–2010.

2. Lymphomas

Lymphoma is the third most common pediatric malignancy - following leukemia and brain tumors - and the most common head and neck cancer in children and adolescents [3]. The broad differential diagnosis for small round blue cell tumors, like lymphoma is shown in **Table 1**. The treatment of childhood lymphoma has experienced significant improvements in recent decades and is now associated with cure rates approaching 80 to 90% [4, 5]. Lymphoma is divided into two groups: Hodgkin lymphoma (HL) and non-Hodgkin lymphoma (NHL). HL is further subdivided into two clinical subtypes by the World Health Organization (WHO) classification which includes classic Hodgkin lymphoma (CHL), which accounts for approximately 95% of HL cases within the United States, and nodular lymphocyte-predominant Hodgkin lymphoma (NLPHL). Overall, HL is less common

Melanoma
Lymphoma
Burkitt lymphoma
Anaplastic large cell lymphoma
Rhabdomyosarcoma
Alveolar
Embryonal
Undifferentiated sarcoma
Ewing Sarcoma
Primitive neuroectodermal tumors (PNET)
Clear cell sarcoma ("melanoma of soft parts")
Neuroendocrine carcinoma
Mesenchymal chondrosarcoma
Sinonasal undifferentiated carcinoma (SNUC)
Nephroblastoma (Wilms tumor)
Retinoblastoma
Neuroblastoma
Hepatoblastoma

Table 1.
Differential diagnosis of small round blue cell tumors.

in developed countries with distribution patterns that vary widely according to geography and ethnicity. HL is characterized by a bimodal distribution with a peak in adolescence between 15 and 40 years of age and another in adulthood beyond 60 years of age. Recently, HL has been shown to cluster within certain families with associations to specific HLA loci, thus suggesting vertical transmission of susceptible genotypes [6]. Pediatric HL exhibits a 2:1 male predominance with as many as 40 to 50% of cases linked to the Epstein Barr virus (EBV) infection as well as the pathognomonic Reed-Sternberg cell morphology [7–9]. Four subtypes of HL have been characterized: nodular sclerosis, mixed cellularity, lymphocyte predominant, and lymphocyte depleted, which account for roughly 50%, 30%, 15%, and less than 10% of the cases, respectively [10]. The Ann Arbor staging system is used to stratify these tumors based on the extent of disease and whether organs on one or both sides of the diaphragm are involved (**Table 2**).

In contrast to HL, the incidence of pediatric NHL is lower in younger children and increases with age. Pediatric NHL is more frequently associated with higher grades and extranodal involvement when compared to cases of adult NHL. Average survival rates are greater than 80%, regardless of histologic subtype, of which there are several [4]. The most common pediatric NHL subtype is Burkitt lymphoma (BL) which accounts for 50 to 60% of childhood cases, followed by T-cell lymphoblastic lymphoma (1520%), anaplastic large cell lymphoma (1015%), diffuse large B-cell lymphoma (510%), followed by other rare subtypes [11]. BL, a highly aggressive tumor, is derived from the classic t(8;14) cytogenetic translocation of the *MYC* oncogene resulting in a constitutive overexpression of c-*myc* leading to rapid cell division [12, 13]. EBV is a well-known endemic oncogenic driver and is most prevalent in regions such as Africa where malaria continues to thrive. Young patients often present with the characteristic mandibular tumor with extranodal and multifocal involvement (in gastrointestinal, hematologic, breast, and ovarian tissues) [14]. Compared to endemic BL, its sporadic form is more common in non-endemic regions such as the United States and Europe [15]. Sporadic form patients are more likely to be male and older (median age 30 years old) with localized lymphadenopathy, large abdominal masses, extranodal disease (2385%), central nervous system involvement (10%), and bone marrow manifestations (13–40%) [16, 17]. Moreover, children with

Stage	Description
I	Involvement of a single lymph node region (cervical, axillary, inguinal, mediastinal) or lymphoid structure (spleen, thymus, or Waldeyer's ring) (I); or extralymphatic site in the absence of involved nodes (I-E)
II	Two or more sites on the same side of the diaphragm (II) including: • Two or more lymph node regions • Regional lymph nodes with associated local lymphoid structure involvement • Extralymphatic site with regional node involvement (II-E)
III	Involvement of regional lymph nodes or lymphoid structures on both sides of the diaphragm (III): • With or without extension to extralymphatic tissue (III-E), the spleen (III-S), or both (III-E,S)
IV	Diffuse or disseminated involvement (IV) of: • One or more extralymphatic organs with or without associated lymph node involvement • Non-contiguous extralymphatic involvement in conjunction with stage II nodal disease • Involvement of the liver, bone marrow, lungs, or cerebrospinal fluid

Table 2.
Ann Arbor staging for Hodgkin lymphoma.

immunodeficiency syndromes or medical treatment for primary malignancies carry an increased risk for developing NHL. Predisposing conditions such as ataxia telangiectasia, Nijmegen syndrome, and various mismatch repair diseases incur not only increased risk of developing NHL but also increase mortality rates from anti-tumor interventions [18]. Immunodeficiency-associated BL is diagnosed in patients with Human Immunodeficiency virus (HIV), though the risk of tumor development declines with the use of antiretroviral therapy [19–21].

Lymphomas of the head and neck can present insidiously, but are typically discovered as a "rubbery," enlarged cervical or supraclavicular lymph node on physical examination. The majority of HL patients present with asymptomatic cervical adenopathy with or without the constitutional "B" symptoms including fever, night sweats, chills and weight loss which are also incorporated into the HL Ann Arbor staging system. While adult NHL is characterized by nodal disease, pediatric NHL has a predisposition for extranodal involvement with the most common head and neck extranodal localizations involving the larynx, sinonasal cavities, salivary glands and orbit. Lymphoma is present within Waldeyer's ring in approximately 44% of cases especially in NHL patients [7, 22]. Oguz et al. conducted a retrospective study of 457 pediatric patients with lymphadenopathy and demonstrated that chronic lymphadenopathy (greater than 4 weeks in duration), generalized and supraclavicular involvement, and lymph nodes measuring greater than 3 cm were findings most commonly associated with malignancy among 111 patients with confirmed disease [23]. Other causes for concern include persistent lymphadenopathy despite antibiosis, nodal firmness, immobility, fixation to underlying tissues, and progressive nodal enlargement [7].

Otolaryngologists and other surgeons primarily serve diagnostic roles via lymph node biopsy As the initial differential diagnosis for pediatric cervical adenopathy is broad and widely varied, a detailed history and physical examination is critical to stratify the likelihood of malignancy against other processes such as infection, hypersensitivity reactions, granulomatous diseases, and rheumatic or lymphoproliferative disorders as these patients may present prior to evaluation by other clinicians. Prior to surgery, management and workup should include an array of laboratory testing which includes complete blood count (CBC) with differential and peripheral blood smear, erythrocyte sedimentation rate (ESR), C-reactive protein (CRP) level, lactate dehydrogenase (LDH), as well as a serum ferritin, copper and alkaline phosphatase levels. Bone marrow biopsy and lumbar puncture (LP) are also routinely performed. Imaging should include chest radiograph and ultrasound (US) with computed tomography and magnetic resonance imaging (MRI) reserved for more suspicious or concerning presentations. Ultrasound is often the imaging mainstay given its accessibility without the need for sedation or radiation exposure (**Table 3**); however, CT continues to play an integral role in surveillance because of simplicity and rapidity. F-fluorodeoxyglucose positron emission tomography (FDG-PET) has demonstrated improved sensitivity and specificity in accurately diagnosing lymphoma compared to conventional imaging modalities [24, 25] (**Figure 2**).

Following imaging, biopsy is needed to obtain a sufficient amount of tissue for frozen and permanent histopathologic analysis along with flow cytometry and immunohistochemistry as indicated. These specimens should be sent fresh rather than in formalin to provide a viable sample responsive to flow cytometry. Following diagnosis, staging of disease typically requires bone marrow biopsy and lumbar puncture to assess extent of bone marrow involvement and to determine whether malignant cells are present in the CSF, respectively. Diagnosis based on fine needle aspiration biopsy (FNAB) has remained controversial and challenging as it results in a dearth of cellularity from sclerosis, decreased detection of clonal populations, and a lack of diagnostic Reed-Sternberg cells [26]. As such, excisional biopsy remains the gold standard in the primary diagnosis of pediatric lymphoma.

	Size	Shape	Borders	Hilar fat, Cortex	Vascular flow[a]	Chronicity	Additional Characteristics
Benign	Typically <2 cm	Long axis to short axis ratio ≥ 2:1; Oval or reniform	Typically blurred, regular	Echogenic, hypoechoic	Hilar (radiating from center), avascular Low vascular resistance	N/A	Calcifications possible
Reactive	Variable	Long axis to short axis ratio ≥ 1:1	Blurred, regular	Echogenic, hypoechoic	Hilar flow, avascular Low vascular resistance	Typically acute (0–2 weeks) or subacute (2–6 weeks)	Calcifications possible
Malignant	Typically >2 cm	Long axis to short axis ratio < 2:1 Round	Typically sharp, irregular. Matting indicates malignancy[b]	Hypoechogenic, hypoechoic	Peripheral flow (cortical), mixed flow Elevated vascular resistance	Chronic, >6 weeks suggests malignancy	Necrosis (cystic or coagulation), calcifications, reticular internal pattern

[a]Hilar (radiating from hilum to cortex), peripheral (flow around cortex); Vascular resistance <0.7 associated with benign process.
[b]Matting: Blending capsules of adjacent lymph nodes.

Table 3.
Ultrasound findings of benign versus malignant head and neck lymph nodes.

Treatment of pediatric lymphoma is non-surgical and includes multi-agent chemotherapy with or without radiotherapy (RT) as the first line. With respect to the treatment of HL, various combinations of chemotherapeutic agents have been utilized with 3- and 8-year event-free survival (EFS) approximating 90% and greater than 80%, respectively, while overall survival (OS) has been demonstrated to range from 80 to 90% [27, 28]. Some regimens include MOPP (mechlorethamine, vincristine, procarbazine, prednisone), COPP (cyclophosphamide, vincristine, procarbazine, prednisone), and ABVD (adriamycin, bleomycin, vinblastine, dacarbazine) [7], each uniquely selected based upon the subtype of HL and the side-effect profiles. RT is also commonly added in combination with

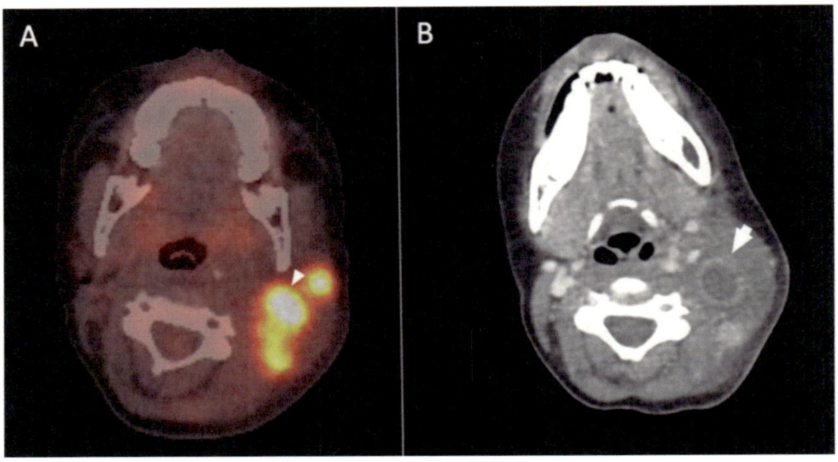

Figure 2.
Axial CT/PET (A) and axial CT neck with contrast (B) of 10-year-old patient with lymphoblastic lymphoma most notable in the left cervical chain. The left jugulodigastric nodes are hypermetabolic (arrowhead) on CT/PET and enlarged with a hypodense central core with rim-enhancement (arrow) on contrasted CT.

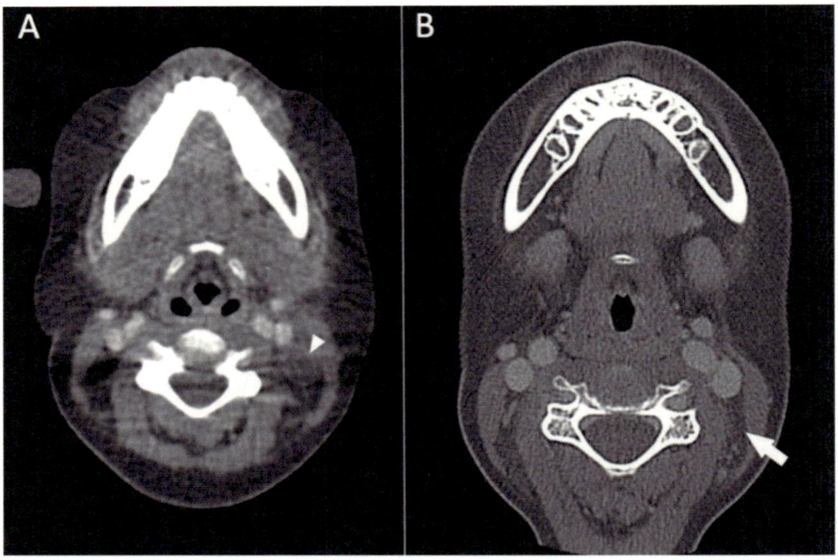

Figure 3.
(A) Axial CT 1 month status post induction chemotherapy for the same patient noted in **Figure 2** *with lymphoblastic lymphoma. Note residual 1.5 cm node (arrowhead). (B) Axial CT scan of the same patient 8 months following diagnosis, following completion of chemotherapy. The previously noted adenopathy has resolved (arrow) and there is no evidence of recurrence.*

chemotherapy. With NHL, a large number of chemotherapeutic combinations are possible, as outlined by Kahn et al.: ABV (doxorubicin, bleomycin, and vinblastine), CHOP (cyclophosphamide, doxorubicin, vincristine, and prednisone) COPDAC (cyclophosphamide, vincristine, prednisone, and dacarbazine), and COPP [29]. In contrast to HL, RT is infrequently used to treat NHL. Additionally, if high-grade NHL is present, intrathecal chemotherapy may be indicated. Post-operative surveillance examinations and imaging are obtained at regular intervals to monitor for evidence of disease recurrence (**Figure 3**).

3. Rhabdomyosarcoma

Rhabdomyosarcoma (RMS), a malignant tumor of mesenchymal origin, is the most common pediatric soft tissue sarcoma affecting approximately 250 children per year within the United States [30]. It accounts for 4.5% of all childhood malignancies and is the third most common extracranial pediatric solid tumor following Wilms' tumor (nephroblastoma) and neuroblastoma. RMS of childhood is characterized by a bimodal distribution and presents between the ages of 2 and 6 and again between 10 and 18 years of age [31]. Although this tumor may arise throughout the body given its mesenchymal nature, the head and neck is the most commonly involved, comprising 35% of all cases [32–34]. Of the cases involving the head and neck, nearly 75% arise within the orbit or parameningeal regions (e.g. nasopharynx, nasal cavity, paranasal sinuses, infratemporal fossa, pterygopalatine fossae, and middle ear) (**Figure 4**). The remainder originates primarily in the oral cavity, cheek, parotid region and soft tissues of the neck, which are commonly referred to as non-orbital or non-parameningeal lesions [35, 36]. Although most tumors occur sporadically, some RMS cases are associated with familial syndromes such as Li Fraumeni and neurofibromatosis type I [31, 37, 38]. The tumor typically presents as a painless, asymptomatic mass in the majority of cases but may cause compressive symptoms and cranial neuropathies secondary to mass effect in more advanced disease.

RMS histology classically appears as a small round blue cell tumor of childhood and is classified alongside similar appearing neoplasms including lymphoma,

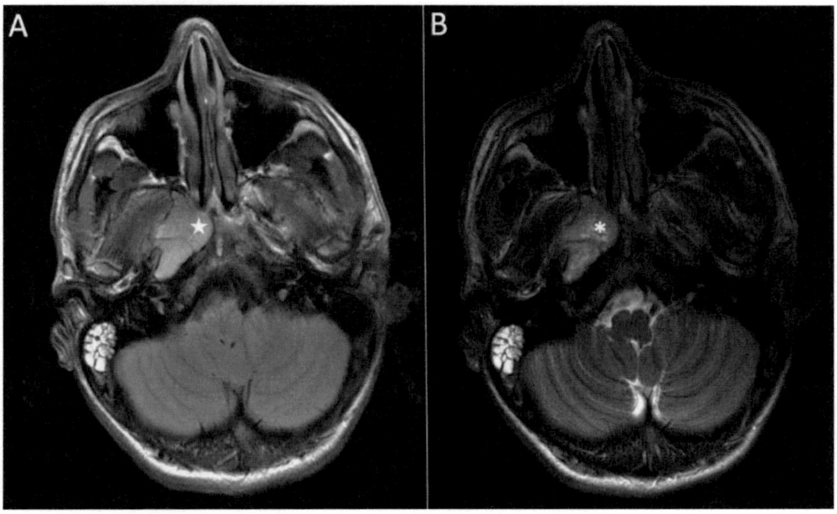

Figure 4.
Embryonal rhabdomyosarcoma. Axial T1 fat-saturated MRI (A) reveals slightly hyper-intense lobular mass of the sphenoid wing (star). Axial T2 MRI (B) reveals the same lesion with similar signal intensity (asterisk).

neuroblastoma, Wilms' tumor, Ewing's sarcoma and peripheral neuroectodermal tumors. There are two main histologic subtypes of RMS: embryonal (ERMS) and alveolar (ARMS). ERMS is the more common subtype and comprises approximately 75% of cases with a preponderance for younger patients. In contrast, the ARMS subtype—appearing histologically similar to pulmonary parenchyma—represents approximately 25% of cases and is more prevalent among older children and adolescents with the majority occurring in children greater than 10 years of age. Compared to ERMS, the ARMS subtype is associated with an unfavorable prognosis. A review of the SEER database performed by Ognjanovic et al. analyzed the incidence and survival rates for pediatric and adolescent RMS between 1975 and 2005 with five-year overall survival rates ranging from 40.1–47.8% and 60.9–73.4% for the ARMS and ERMS types, respectively [39]. Similar findings were reported by Pappo et al. with five-year survival rates of 97% for non-orbital, non-parameningeal embryonal cases versus 67% for ARMS subtypes [35]. With respect to head and neck tumors, the ERMS subtype occurs more frequently and may be further classified into the botryoid and spindle-cell variants with botryoid histology demonstrating a more favorable prognosis [34].

Patients with suspected RMS should undergo a thorough workup including a complete head and neck physical exam along with laboratory testing, imaging and pathologic confirmation prior to treatment. Evaluation for metastatic disease often includes a lumbar puncture for cerebrospinal fluid analysis. Imaging studies of the primary tumor site often involve CT - which is useful for the evaluation of osseous erosion - and MRI for further characterization of the primary tumor and the surrounding anatomy. This is especially beneficial in determining whether the tumor may be safely resected with primary surgery or if neoadjuvant treatment is required to decrease the morbidity. FDG-PET imaging has so far seen limited use in the pediatric population. However, several studies have suggested an increased utility in evaluating the presence of lymphadenopathy, occult disease, response to treatment, and detection of recurrence compared to standard imaging alone [40–43]. Biopsy is required for definitive diagnosis and may often be achieved via fine needle aspiration or open biopsy while taking care to obtain an adequate amount of tissue for accurate histopathologic analysis. Although lymph node involvement in pediatric head and neck RMS is uncommon, determining the presence of locoregional and metastatic lymph node involvement is critical in establishing pre-treatment staging and, in cases of suspected disease, pathologic evaluation should be undertaken which will further influence radiotherapy fields. In an analysis of regional lymph node disease in 898 patients within the pivotal Intergroup Rhabdomyosarcoma Study IV, Rodeberg and colleagues demonstrated that the presence of nodal disease is an independently poor prognostic indicator for both failure-free and overall survival, further underlining the need to establish the extent of disease prior to treatment [44].

In an effort to design effective and tailored treatment regimens for these patients, the Intergroup Rhabdomyosarcoma Study and its subsequent iterations (IRS I-IV) established a staging and grouping system to aid in directing treatment strategy based upon tumor location, disease extent, and completeness of surgical resection [45–48]. Within this classification scheme, the pre-operative "stage" is based upon pre-operative standard TNM staging guidelines whereas the post-operative clinical "group" refers to the extent of disease and completeness of surgical resection prior to adjuvant therapy. Group I reflects complete resection with negative pathologic margins. Group II consists of patients with complete gross resection but microscopically positive residual disease (close or positive margins, presence of regional nodal disease, or both). Group III includes patients with gross residual disease following incomplete resection or unresectable disease. Group IV reflects those with distant metastatic disease other than first echelon nodal metastases.

An overview of the IRS pre-treatment staging (**Tables 4** and **5**) and post-treatment grouping classification (**Table 6**) is provided.

Chemotherapy and radiation have remained the mainstay of multimodal treatment for childhood RMS. Recently, there has been an increasing trend towards

Stage	Sites	T	Tumor size	N	M
I	Orbit	T1 or T2	a or b	N0, N1, or Nx	M0
	Head and neck (excluding parameningeal)		a or b	N0, N1, or Nx	
	Genitourinary (non-bladder/non-prostate)		a or b	N0, N1, or Nx	
II	Bladder/prostate	T1 or T2	a	N0 or Nx	M0
	Extremity		a	N0 or Nx	
	Head and neck (parameningeal)		a	N0 or Nx	
	Other (includes trunk, retroperitoneum, etc.)		a	N0 or Nx	
III	Bladder/Prostate	T1 or T2	a	N1	M0
	Extremity		b	N0, N1, or Nx	
	Head and neck (parameningeal)		b	N0, N1, or Nx	
	Other (includes trunk, retroperitoneum, etc.)		b	N0, N1, or Nx	
IV	All	T1 or T2	a or b	N0 or Nx	M1

Table 4.
TNM pre-treatment staging system for rhabdomyosarcoma.

Classification	Description
Tumor	
T1	Confined to anatomic site of origin
a	<5 cm in diameter
b	≥5 cm in diameter
T2	Extension and/or fixation to surrounding tissue
a	<5 cm in diameter
b	≥5 cm in diameter
Regional lymph nodes	
N0	Not clinically involved
N1	Clinically involved
Nx	Clinical status unknown
Metastases	
M0	No distant metastases
M1	Distant metastases present

Table 5.
Pre-treatment rhabdomyosarcoma TNM classifications.

Clinical Group	Criteria
Group 1	Localized disease, complete resection, no microscopic residual disease
A	Confined to site of origin, complete resection
B	Infiltrating beyond site of origin, complete resection
Group 2	Gross total resection
A	Gross resection with microscopic residual disease
B	Regional disease with spread to regional lymph nodes, complete resection without residual microscopic disease
C	Regional disease with spread to regional lymph nodes, gross total resection, but evidence of microscopic residual disease
Group 3	Incomplete resection or biopsy with gross residual disease remaining
Group 4	Distant metastases present irrespective of surgical approach to tumor

Table 6.
Post-surgical clinical group staging system for rhabdomyosarcoma.

primary surgical resection in localized tumors involving the head and neck [49]. The success of surgical treatment is often dependent on the specific location of tumor [35, 36, 50, 51]. Orbital RMS, associated with a favorable prognosis, is rarely associated with meningeal extension and is treated with primary chemotherapy and radiation with surgery reserved for salvage cases [52]. On the other hand, parameningeal lesions are more challenging to remove and are often categorized as IRS Group III tumors because they are not typically amenable to complete surgical resection. Given its anatomic location in close proximity to vital neurovascular structures, parameningeal RMS is associated with an increased likelihood of cranial neuropathies, cranial base erosion, and intracranial extension [53]. As primary surgical resection with wide margins is often infeasible for these tumors, chemotherapy with or without radiation is the preferred treatment modalities. (**Figures 4** and **5**). Reilly et al. conducted a retrospective chart review of 17 children diagnosed with head and neck RMS over an 18-year period and found that the majority presented with cranial neuropathies, thus reflecting the aggressive nature of this disease upon symptom

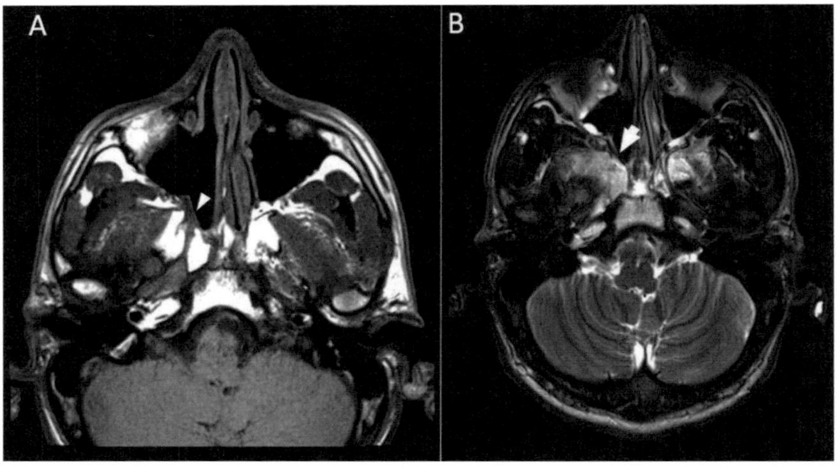

Figure 5.
Axial T1 MRI (A) performed 18 months after biopsy, chemotherapy, and proton therapy to treat embryonal rhabdomyosarcoma noted in **Figure 4** *with no evidence of recurrence at the primary site (arrowhead). Axial T2 MRI (B) of the same patient at 39 months post-treatment, still with no evidence of recurrence (arrow).*

onset with 5 of 17 (29.4%) patients demonstrating advanced metastatic disease at first referral. Within their series, 4 of 4 patients with non-parameningeal disease underwent primary surgical resection but tumor-free margins were unobtainable and adjuvant chemotherapy with radiation was ultimately required. All patients with parameningeal disease underwent multimodal treatment [54]. However, Daya et al. also demonstrated that many children may avoid radiation therapy without compromising survival in cases of completely resected RMS [49].

In general, pediatric RMS necessitates systemic treatment in the form of chemotherapy with local control achieved with surgery and/or radiation. The treatment approach must nonetheless be carefully tailored for each individual patient according to tumor location and the potential morbidities associated with each modality. Although primary surgical resection may be possible in select non-parameningeal tumors, the decision for adjuvant therapy is ultimately determined by margin status.

4. Thyroid carcinoma

Thyroid carcinoma represents approximately 21% of all pediatric head and neck malignancies with an annual reported incidence of 0.54 per 100,000 persons within the United States [55, 56]. In contrast to adults, thyroid nodules are less likely to be palpable in children (2% vs. 35%) and carry a much higher likelihood of malignancy with a risk of 1 in 4 in pediatric patients compared to less than 1 in 10 for adults [57]. The majority of thyroid cancers are differentiated with papillary thyroid cancer (PTC) accounting for greater than 90% of cases [56]. Less common variants include follicular thyroid cancer (FTC) and medullary thyroid cancer (MTC) while anaplastic and poorly differentiated subtypes are even rarer [58]. MTC is more common among younger children (ages 0–4) and declines with increasing age while the incidence of PTC increases as one approaches adolescence and adulthood [55]. A significant number of patients present with regional lymph node involvement (60–80%) and distant metastatic disease may occur in up to 20% of children with the lungs most commonly involved [59]. Despite the frequency of advanced disease at initial presentation, several case series have demonstrated an excellent prognosis with greater than 95% long-term survival for papillary and follicular variants [58, 60–62]. Notably, previous radiation exposure and treatment of other childhood malignancies increases the risk for developing pediatric thyroid cancer with an 18-fold greater risk of thyroid cancer compared to the general population, thus highlighting the importance of close follow up and frequent surveillance among this cohort [63–65].

The diagnosis of suspected pediatric thyroid cancer involves a focused history and physical examination with particular attention to previous radiation exposure and treatment of prior childhood malignancies, such as lymphoma. Patients typically present with an asymptomatic thyroid nodule or mass following incidental discovery on surveillance imaging studies. US and FNAB of the most suspicious thyroid nodules should be completed along with histocytologic analysis. A review of 89 pediatric patients by Buryk et al. examined patients with thyroid nodules ≥0.8 cm and demonstrated that larger-sized nodules, palpable nodules, and palpable lymphadenopathy were significant predictors of malignancy [66]. Sonographic characteristics associated with malignant nodules include larger size, solid parenchyma, taller-than-wide shape, microcalcifications, irregular margins, and abnormal-appearing lymph nodes [67–69]. Richman et al. also found significantly increased rates of cancer in patients with solitary nodules compared to those with multiple nodules (29.4% vs. 14.2%, $p = 0.003$) [69]. Although US is essential characterizing thyroid lesions, results may vary according to sonographer skill. Neck and chest CT may be useful in evaluating for metastatic disease, cervical lymphadenopathy, and in surgical planning, especially in cases with large-volume or bulky disease. Laboratory testing is particularly important and should include thyroid-stimulating hormone (TSH), T3, and T4 levels. Serum calcitonin level should also be obtained in any patient with known or suspected multiple endocrine neoplasia (MEN) syndrome, although routine use remains controversial in patients with seemingly isolated MTC [70]. Genetic testing and referral should be considered in familial cases and in patients with confirmed MTC or MEN syndrome.

Surgical resection is the primary treatment modality for childhood thyroid cancer with options including total thyroidectomy and lobectomy with isthmusectomy. The American Thyroid Association (ATA) guidelines utilize the American Joint Committee on Cancer (AJCC) pTMN staging system to stratify patients into low, intermediate, and high-risk groups. Total thyroidectomy is the preferred surgical method for PTC given an increased likelihood of bilateral and multifocal disease in these tumors [71] (**Table 7**). The extent of resection nonetheless remains a source of controversy. Nice et al. performed a retrospective review of 3861 patients less than 21 years old with primary PTC nodule greater than 1 cm in diameter and found no significant difference between total thyroidectomy compared to partial thyroidectomy (e.g. sublobar resection, lobectomy, or lobectomy with isthmusectomy) on both univariate and multivariate analyses, with both groups demonstrating

ATA risk level	Definition[a]	Initial post-operative staging[b]	Surveillance for pediatric patients with no evidence of disease
Low	Disease grossly confined to the thyroid with N0/Nx disease or Disease grossly confined to the thyroid with N0/Nx disease (microscopic metastases to a small number of central neck lymph nodes)	Tg[c]	US at 6 months postoperatively, then annually x 5 years Tg[c] on LT_4 every 3–6 months x 2 years, then annually
Intermediate	Extensive N1a or minimal N1b disease	TSH-stimulated Tg[c] and diagnostic ^{123}I scan	US at 6 months postoperatively, every 6–12 months x 5 years, then less frequently Tg[c] on LT_4 every 3–6 months x 3 years, then annually Consider TSH-stimulated Tg[c] ± diagnostic ^{123}I scan in 1–2 years in patients previously treated with ^{131}I
High	Regionally extensive disease (extensive N1b) or Locally invasive disease (T4 tumors), with or without distant metastasis	TSH-stimulated Tg[c] and diagnostic ^{123}I scan	US at 6 months postoperatively, every 6–12 months x 5 years, then less frequently Tg[c] on LT_4 every 3–6 months x 3 years, then annually Consider TSH-stimulated Tg[c] ± diagnostic ^{123}I scan in 1–2 years in patients previously treated with ^{131}I

[a] *TNM staging from the AJCC Cancer Staging Manual, 7th edition.*
[b] *Completed within 12 weeks following surgery.*
[c] *Assumes the absence of thyroglobulin autoantibodies.*
LT_4, levothyroxine.

Table 7.
American Thyroid Association (ATA) pediatric thyroid cancer risk classification and post-operative management for papillary thyroid carcinoma in children.

96% 15-year overall survival (OS) [72]. In contrast, Bargen et al. found that, while there were no significant increase in surgical complications, patients receiving less than total thyroidectomy were at an increased risk for requiring revision surgery ($p = 0.03$) [73]. Despite these differences, outcomes for PTC are excellent with long-term survival rates greater than 95% [56, 58, 60–62]. Unlike PTC, FTC is more likely to be unifocal and metastasize via hematogenous spread. FTC is commonly managed with thyroid lobectomy, but total thyroidectomy with radioactive iodine ablation (RAI) is indicated in cases of metastasis, advanced disease, vascular invasion, or extracapsular extension. Selective neck dissection, particularly central node dissection, is recommended for clinically involved or radiographically abnormal lymph nodes, extrathyroidal tumor extension, and evidence of locoregional disease [71]. The utility of neck dissection in the absence of clear clinical indications remains poorly defined, but prophylactic neck dissection may be performed in patients with advanced disease [74].

MTC is a unique variant of thyroid carcinoma. Most pediatric cases are inherited in an autosomal-dominant fashion although sporadic cases are possible. Pediatric MTC patients commonly present with bilateral and multifocal thyroid nodules, with metastatic disease common at the time of diagnosis. Parafollicular C-cell hyperplasia results in an excess production of calcitonin and carcinoembryonic antigen (CEA). Mutations in the *RET* proto-oncogene are responsible for the development of the multiple endocrine neoplasia 2 (MEN 2) syndrome which is divided into three distinct entities based on the endocrine tissues involved: MEN-2A, MEN-2B, and familial MTC [75]. MEN-2A (exons 10 and 11 mutations) is characterized by MTC, pheochromocytoma, and primary hyperparathyroidism from the presence of parathyroid adenomas. MEN-2B (exon 16 mutations) involves MTC, pheochromocytoma, mucosal neuromas (with predisposition for the lips and tongue), ganglioneuromas, and marfanoid body habitus. Familial MTC, a variant of MEN-2A which accounts for 15% of hereditary MTCs, is characterized by a strong familial predisposition to MTC without pheochromocytoma and parathyroid adenomas [76, 77]. In suspected cases, thyroid US and FNAB should be performed. In addition to thyroid function studies, serum calcitonin and CEA levels should be obtained. If concern exists for pheochromocytoma, metanephrine and catecholamine testing should be included along with the imaging studies. Genetic testing is indicated for children with a familial history of *RET* mutations and allows for close surveillance in these patients prior to the development of disease. Prophylactic total thyroidectomy with or without central lymph node dissection is the surgical treatment of choice and may be performed safely in children as early as 5 years of age with a family history of germline RET mutations or MEN-2A syndrome [78–80]. For those with the MEN-2B syndrome, prophylactic thyroidectomy before age 1 may be appropriate, especially if patients are carriers of aggressive codon mutations [81]. There is no clear consensus regarding central neck dissection, although this is often performed at the time of prophylactic total thyroidectomy [71, 74, 82, 83]. The five-year OS for MTC is similarly high at approximately 96%, but, the 15- and 30-year survival rates are lower at 86% [55].

Following total thyroidectomy, hormone replacement is necessary. Together with RAI therapy, it may reduce the risk of tumor recurrence. Long-term surveillance includes serum thyroglobulin levels, thyroid US, and radioiodine-123 (^{123}I) diagnostic whole-body scans. Radioiodine-131 (^{131}I) may be used for ablation of residual thyroid tissue and is indicated in select pediatric patients with distant metastases or residual disease not amenable to surgical resection [71, 84, 85]. Complications of RAI are dose-dependent and include pulmonary fibrosis, infertility, and the development of secondary cancers, thus highlighting the importance of careful patient selection as well as follow-up [86].

5. Nasopharyngeal carcinoma

Nasopharyngeal carcinoma (NPC) is a rare pediatric malignancy. Overall, NPC accounts for less than 1% of all childhood cancers and represents approximately 20–50% of nasopharyngeal tumors [87, 88]. Globally, the incidence of pediatric NPC is highest throughout southeast Asia, southern China, and the Mediterranean. In the United States, childhood NPC is more commonly diagnosed in the southern states. The age distribution is bimodal with the first peak in adolescence followed by mid-adulthood (ages 40–60) while the distribution in endemic regions (e.g. Southeastern Asia and China) is unimodal without a pediatric peak [89]. In all regions, the etiology and pathogenesis of NPC is closely related to Epstein–Barr virus (EBV) infection with children sharing a closer association with EBV than adults [88, 90].

The WHO separates three distinct histopathologic subtypes of NPC: Type I (keratinizing squamous cell carcinoma), Type II (non-keratinizing epidermoid carcinoma), and Type III (undifferentiated carcinoma) (**Table 8**) [88, 91]. Type I is characterized by the production of keratin, is commonly associated with alcohol and tobacco exposure and, as such, is less common in the pediatric population. Type I NPC may be found in those with EBV infections in endemic areas. Type II and III commonly demonstrate lymphoid, plasmoid, and eosinophilic cell infiltration. Type III, also referred to as lymphoepithelioma or Schminke tumor, is the most common histopathologic subtype in pediatric patients and may be found in as many as 90% of patients with a high rate of distant metastases [88].

Childhood NPC most commonly presents a painless neck mass, which may be appreciated in 70–90% of patients at the time of first diagnosis. Nasal obstruction, epistaxis, and Eustachian tube dysfunction with resultant conductive hearing loss and serous otitis media may occur from tumor mass effect [92]. In more advanced disease, trismus, headache, facial pain, diplopia with vision changes, and other cranial nerve palsies may be present secondary to skull base involvement [88, 93, 94]. Patients with systemic disease may present with paraneoplastic syndromes such as syndrome of inappropriate antidiuretic hormone (SIADH) or dermatomyositis [95]. Evaluation involves a thorough clinical examination with contrast-enhanced CT and MRI with particular attention to skull base structures. Recommended laboratory testing includes a CBC, serum chemistry, lactic acid dehydrogenase (LDH) level, and liver function panel. More specifically, elevated LDH levels carry prognostic significance with higher values shown to correlate with decreased OS, disease-free survival (DFS), and distant metastasis-free survival (DMFS) [96, 97]. Bone marrow biopsy and CSF cytologic analysis is indicated in cases of distant metastases or when skull base extension is suspected while biopsy of the primary tumor is required for accurate tissue diagnosis.

Given the rarity of pediatric NPCs, treatment strategies have been tailored from established adult guidelines. As these tumors are rarely amenable to surgical resection, the standard of care for locoregional NPC involves a combination of high-dose

Type	Description
I	Keratinizing squamous cell carcinoma
II	Non-keratinizing carcinoma
III	Undifferentiated carcinoma (Lymphoepithelioma or Schminke tumor)

Table 8.
World Health Organization (WHO) classification of nasopharyngeal carcinoma.

radiotherapy (RT) to the primary nasopharyngeal tumor bed and the surrounding nodal basin with lower doses targeted at surrounding tissues and uninvolved lymph nodes. Due to high rates of locoregional and distant failure in patients presenting with advanced disease, chemotherapeutic regimens have recently been incorporated into treatment schemas. With combined RT and chemotherapy, survival rates ranging from 60 to 70% have been reported with some studies documenting as high as 90% [89, 90, 94, 98, 99]. In patients with early-stage T1 or T2 disease, single modality RT may be utilized. In locally advanced cases, dual modality treatment has been shown to result in improved OS compared to RT alone. A meta-analysis by Langendijk et al. demonstrated that concurrent chemotherapy was associated with a pooled hazard ratio (HR) of 0.48 (95% CI, 0.32–0.72) which corresponded to a 20% improvement in five-year OS compared to RT alone while neoadjuvant chemotherapy was associated with improved locoregional control with a decreased rate of distant metastases [100]. Similar results have been documented throughout the literature [101–105]. Despite these advances, many patients continue to present with locoregional or systemic recurrence with most relapses occurring within the first two years (median 8 months) following treatment [98, 106, 107]. The short interval between therapy completion and distant metastases may be a result of occult disease at the time of presentation. Notably, T and N classification, total irradiation dose, presence of metastatic disease at diagnosis, and delay in time to RT have all been demonstrated as prognostic factors in locoregional control of NPC [93, 105–110].

6. Salivary gland malignancy

Pediatric salivary gland malignancies are rare and comprise approximately 3% of head and neck cancers in the pediatric population and 5% of salivary gland malignancies overall [111]. In contrast to adults, the majority of salivary gland neoplasms in children are malignant in nature (40–60%) and most are epithelial in origin. The parotid gland is the most common site and mucoepidermoid carcinoma (MEC) represents the vast majority of salivary gland malignancies. Less common histologic subtypes include acinic cell carcinoma (24–40%) and adenoid cystic carcinoma (15–26%) [112]. Several series have evaluated treatment outcomes associated with these tumors and demonstrate surgical resection as the mainstay of treatment followed by adjuvant RT in select instances [112–119]. A retrospective study by Ribeiro and colleagues reviewed outcomes associated with the treatment of 38 pediatric patients with salivary gland neoplasms, 27 (71.1%) of whom presented with malignant tumors [116]. MEC was the most frequent pathology occurring in 17 of 27 (69.3%) cases followed by 3 patients with adenoid cystic carcinoma; the remaining seven patients had a diverse range of rare malignancies. The parotid gland was the most common primary site followed by minor salivary glands and submandibular gland with 74.1%, 22.2%, and 7.4% of the cases, respectively. All were treated with surgical resection while 10 patients underwent concurrent neck dissection; however, only 6 were found to have pathologically positive lymph node disease. RT was administered to a total of 10 patients (neoadjuvant in 2 patients, adjuvant in 8 patients) and chemotherapy in 3 individuals. Overall, five and ten-year survival rates were both 81.6% with tumor differentiation found to be a significant prognostic factor in those with MEC with a five-year OS of 100% in low-grade histology compared to 50% for intermediate and high-grade histology ($p = 0.01$). Similar findings have been reported throughout the literature [118–121]. Despite the limited sample size in these series, the results highlight the central role of surgery in these patients with favorable long-term outcomes and facial nerve preservation. Moreover, while adjuvant therapy is utilized in select cases, no standard criteria has been agreed upon likely owing to the relative rarity of these tumors. The decision to pursue RT and chemotherapy varies between institutions with some centers advocating its use in high-grade histology and in the presence of aggressive histological features such as perineural or intravascular invasion; however, soft-tissue extension and multi-level lymph node involvement are findings which more commonly result in its use [118, 119].

While MEC is the most common adult and childhood malignant salivary gland tumor, it has also been reported to occur more frequently in patients previously treated with RT and/or chemotherapy regimens for both cancerous and benign pathology [122–124]. A literature review by Verma et al. assessed the characteristics and treatment outcomes of 58 patients selected from 23 studies with treatment-related MEC and showed a significantly shorter latent time to the development of MEC from initial treatment in those treated with chemotherapy with or without RT compared to RT alone (7.9 years vs. 27.2 years) [120]. The primary MEC treatment modality was surgery alone in the majority of patients (64.9%) or in combination with radiation (29.8%) while the remaining patients received surgery plus chemotherapy, or underwent RT alone. Survival was similar to those documented in previous studies with two and five-year OS rates of 98.0% and 93.4%, respectively. Despite favorable survival, the potential for the development of secondary malignancy underscores the importance of continued surveillance in these patients for not only salivary gland cancers but other solid tumor malignancies (**Table 1**).

Clinically, most salivary gland neoplasms present as asymptomatic masses and are rarely associated with cranial neuropathies; the presence of facial nerve weakness or other cranial nerve deficits should heighten the suspicion for malignant potential [111, 112, 125, 126]. US remains the first-line imaging modality and has been shown to be useful in combination with FNAB in establishing a timely diagnosis, specifically in parotid tumors [127]. While CT is useful for further imaging characterization, MRI is superior in demonstrating soft-tissue enhancement which is particularly beneficial in evaluating the status of the facial nerve, lingual nerve, and other surrounding neurovascular structures [128]. Open biopsy should be avoided given the potential for injury to the facial nerve, especially in children with parotid tumors, and possibility for tumor seeding [129, 130]. Treatment consists of local excision with tumor-free margins of the affected salivary gland. In the case of partial or total parotidectomy, careful attention to preserving facial nerve function is recommended as the critical neurovascular structures are smaller in pediatric patients. The same principles hold true in cases of submandibular gland malignancy where the marginal mandibular and lingual nerve should be preserved [112, 131]. A review of the SEER database from 1973 to 2006 by Sultan et al. identified a total of 263 children and adolescents with salivary gland carcinoma and, in comparison to adults, found that disease is more often localized (50%) with regional lymph node metastases being less common (11% vs. 31%) [117]. The need for neck dissection in children is poorly understood as the majority of tumors are low-grade without occult nodal disease. As a result, several authors have suggested that neck dissection be performed in cases of clinically evident nodal involvement and high-grade histology which may altogether avoid the need for adjuvant therapy in the absence of positive margins or pathologically positive nodal disease [116, 125, 132, 133].

7. Osteosarcoma

Sarcomas account for 14% of primary head and neck malignancies in children and adolescents. Osteosarcoma remains the most common subtype consisting of approximately 0.5% of the cases and Ewing sarcoma is the second most common cancer of bone [1]. Osteosarcoma most frequently involves the long bones of the extremities (e.g. distal femur, proximal tibia, proximal humerus) but may occur in the mandible or maxilla which are the most commonly involved head and neck subsites [134–139]. In general, childhood mandibular and maxillary tumors are benign and are discovered incidentally during routine dental examinations or non-related imaging studies [140, 141]. Head and neck osteosarcoma is also associated with a better prognosis when compared to their long bone counterparts with three and five-year survival rate at approximately 65% [142–144]. Patients tend to present during adolescence with a painless mandibular mass, but pain, edema, loose dentition, paresthesias, diplopia, or cranial nerve palsies are especially suspicious for malignancy [134, 135, 144].

Management and treatment protocols are primarily based upon large trials or meta-analyses focused on osteosarcoma of the limbs and trunk [145]. In addition to laboratory studies, imaging commonly involves a combination of plain radiographs, CT, MRI, and 99 m technetium methylene disphosphonate bone scans [146–148]. The classic "sunburst" finding in addition to a "fluffy" or spiculated osseous appearance suggests the presence of an aggressive periosteal reaction along with osteolytic or osteoblastic bony destruction associated with malignancy. Lesions are sampled for histologic determination of subtype which includes the osteoblastic, chondroblastic, and fibroblastic high-grade forms with tumor grade carrying prognostic significance [137, 149–152]. Estimating survival rates for pediatric head and neck osteosarcoma is difficult as studies tend to group adult and pediatric patients together. Despite this, surgical resection appears to play an important role with negative surgical margins being the most important prognostic factor [142, 143, 153–157]. Similar to other surgically resected tumors, adjuvant RT and chemotherapy are reserved for use in cases with incompletely resected disease or in the setting of positive surgical margins. In the case of unresectable disease, RT and chemotherapy either as single or multi-modal therapy may be indicated,

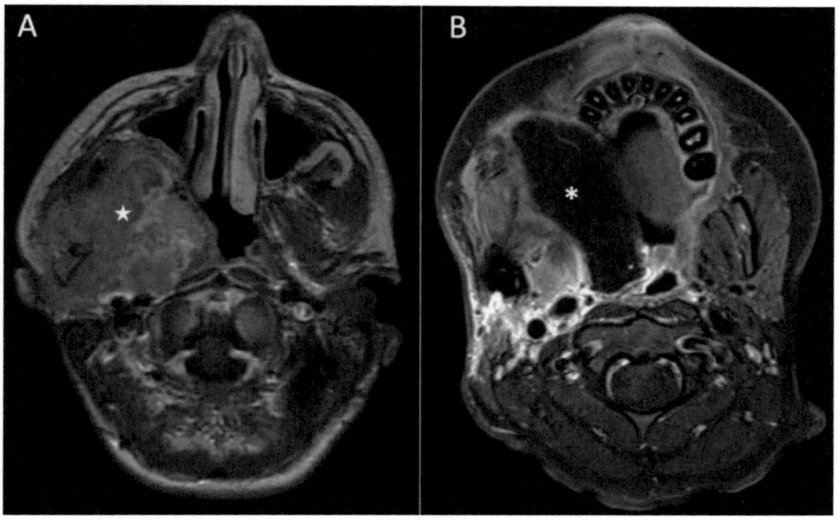

Figure 6.
Monophasic synovial sarcoma. (A) Post-contrast axial T1 MRI demonstrating a T4aN0M0 monophasic synovial cell sarcoma of the right infratemporal fossa and parapharyngeal space in a 15-year-old male (star). Post-contrast axial T1 fat suppressed MRI (B) status-post composite resection demonstrating a right segmental mandibulectomy and resection of tumor involving the infratemporal fossa, parapharyngeal space, and pterygoid base. A total parotidectomy with facial nerve preservation and right selective neck dissection (levels I-IV) was also performed. The 1-month postoperative fibula free flap is visualized (asterisk).

though RT should be approached with particular care as some studies attribute RT as a causative intervention for OS. Other less common sarcomas exist (e.g., fibrosarcoma, synovial cell sarcoma, chondrosarcoma, liposarcoma), although a complete discussion of the management of these entities is outside the scope of this review. Nonetheless, surgical resection remains the mainstay of treatment in many of these diagnoses and leads to a successful outcome when complete resection with tumor-free margins is obtained (**Figure 6**).

8. Conclusion

Pediatric head and neck malignancies represent a minority of childhood tumors. Although the relative rarity of these tumors largely prevents initiation of high-volume trials, experiences from adult cases and in pediatric case reports stipulate that multimodal therapy is often indicated based upon the specific histopathology, stage, and anatomic sites involved. In select instances, primary surgical management with or without free tissue transfer and microvascular reconstruction may also be indicated. While adjuvant therapy including post-operative radiation may improve long-term survival rates, careful consideration must be given to the potential for the development of deleterious side effects in young children including secondary malignancies later in life.

Acknowledgements

This research did not receive any specific grant from funding agencies in the public, commercial, or not-for-profit sectors.

Conflict of interest

The authors declare no relevant conflicts of interest.

Author details

Dustin A. Silverman[1], Ross Wanner[2], Patrick Walz[1], Matthew O. Old[3] and Kris R. Jatana[1*]

1 Department of Otolaryngology – Head and Neck Surgery, Nationwide Children's Hospital and Wexner Medical Center at Ohio State University, Columbus, OH, USA

2 The Ohio State University College of Medicine, Columbus, OH, USA

3 Division of Head and Neck Oncology, Department of Otolaryngology - Head and Neck Surgery, Wexner Medical Center at Ohio State University, James Cancer Center and Solove Research Institute, Columbus, OH, USA

*Address all correspondence to: kris.jatana@nationwidechildrens.org

References

[1] Albright JT, Topham AK, Reilly JS. Pediatric head and neck malignancies: US incidence and trends over 2 decades. Archives of otolaryngology--head & neck surgery. 2002;128:655-9.

[2] Choi DK, Helenowski I, Hijiya N. Secondary malignancies in pediatric cancer survivors: perspectives and review of the literature. International journal of cancer. 2014;135:1764-73.

[3] Linabery AM, Ross JA. Trends in childhood cancer incidence in the U.S. (1992-2004). Cancer. 2008;112:416-32.

[4] Minard-Colin V, Brugieres L, Reiter A, Cairo MS, Gross TG, Woessmann W, et al. Non-Hodgkin Lymphoma in Children and Adolescents: Progress Through Effective Collaboration, Current Knowledge, and Challenges Ahead. Journal of clinical oncology : official journal of the American Society of Clinical Oncology. 2015;33:2963-74.

[5] Gross TG, Termuhlen AM. Pediatric non-Hodgkin's lymphoma. Current oncology reports. 2007;9:459-65.

[6] Kharazmi E, Fallah M, Pukkala E, Olsen JH, Tryggvadottir L, Sundquist K, et al. Risk of familial classical Hodgkin lymphoma by relationship, histology, age, and sex: a joint study from five Nordic countries. Blood. 2015;126:1990-5.

[7] Gaini RM, Romagnoli M, Sala A, Garavello W. Lymphomas of head and neck in pediatric patients. International journal of pediatric otorhinolaryngology. 2009;73 Suppl 1:S65-70.

[8] Weiner MA, Leventhal BG, Marcus R, Brecher M, Ternberg J, Behm FG, et al. Intensive chemotherapy and low-dose radiotherapy for the treatment of advanced-stage Hodgkin's disease in pediatric patients: a Pediatric Oncology Group study. Journal of clinical oncology : official journal of the American Society of Clinical Oncology. 1991;9:1591-8.

[9] Linabery AM, Erhardt EB, Fonstad RK, Ambinder RF, Bunin GR, Ross JA, et al. Infectious, autoimmune and allergic diseases and risk of Hodgkin lymphoma in children and adolescents: a Children's Oncology Group study. International journal of cancer. 2014;135:1454-69.

[10] Donaldson SS. Pediatric Hodgkin's disease--up, up, and beyond. Int J Radiat Oncol Biol Phys. 2002;54:1-8.

[11] Burkhardt B, Zimmermann M, Oschlies I, Niggli F, Mann G, Parwaresch R, et al. The impact of age and gender on biology, clinical features and treatment outcome of non-Hodgkin lymphoma in childhood and adolescence. Br J Haematol. 2005;131:39-49.

[12] Casulo C, Friedberg JW. Burkitt lymphoma- a rare but challenging lymphoma. Best practice & research Clinical haematology. 2018;31:279-84.

[13] Dave SS, Fu K, Wright GW, Lam LT, Kluin P, Boerma EJ, et al. Molecular diagnosis of Burkitt's lymphoma. The New England journal of medicine. 2006;354:2431-42.

[14] Blum KA, Lozanski G, Byrd JC. Adult Burkitt leukemia and lymphoma. Blood. 2004;104:3009-20.

[15] Morton LM, Wang SS, Devesa SS, Hartge P, Weisenburger DD, Linet MS. Lymphoma incidence patterns by WHO subtype in the United States, 1992-2001. Blood. 2006;107:265-76.

[16] Hoelzer D, Walewski J, Dohner H, Viardot A, Hiddemann W,

Spiekermann K, et al. Improved outcome of adult Burkitt lymphoma/ leukemia with rituximab and chemotherapy: report of a large prospective multicenter trial. Blood. 2014;124:3870-9.

[17] Mead GM, Sydes MR, Walewski J, Grigg A, Hatton CS, Pescosta N, et al. An international evaluation of CODOX-M and CODOX-M alternating with IVAC in adult Burkitt's lymphoma: results of United Kingdom Lymphoma Group LY06 study. Annals of oncology : official journal of the European Society for Medical Oncology. 2002;13:1264-74.

[18] Attarbaschi A, Carraro E, Abla O, Barzilai-Birenboim S, Bomken S, Brugieres L, et al. Non-Hodgkin lymphoma and pre-existing conditions: spectrum, clinical characteristics and outcome in 213 children and adolescents. Haematologica. 2016;101:1581-91.

[19] Barta SK, Samuel MS, Xue X, Wang D, Lee JY, Mounier N, et al. Changes in the influence of lymphoma- and HIV-specific factors on outcomes in AIDS-related non-Hodgkin lymphoma. Annals of oncology : official journal of the European Society for Medical Oncology. 2015;26:958-66.

[20] Simcock M, Blasko M, Karrer U, Bertisch B, Pless M, Blumer L, et al. Treatment and prognosis of AIDS-related lymphoma in the era of highly active antiretroviral therapy: findings from the Swiss HIV Cohort Study. Antiviral therapy. 2007;12:931-9.

[21] Gabarre J, Raphael M, Lepage E, Martin A, Oksenhendler E, Xerri L, et al. Human immunodeficiency virus-related lymphoma: relation between clinical features and histologic subtypes. The American journal of medicine. 2001;111:704-11.

[22] Shen Y. [Clinical analysis of non-Hodgkin lymphoma of the head and neck (report of 25 cases)]. Lin chuang er bi yan hou ke za zhi = Journal of clinical otorhinolaryngology. 2005;19:311-2.

[23] Oguz A, Karadeniz C, Temel EA, Citak EC, Okur FV. Evaluation of peripheral lymphadenopathy in children. Pediatric hematology and oncology. 2006;23:549-61.

[24] Kluge R, Kurch L, Georgi T, Metzger M. Current Role of FDG-PET in Pediatric Hodgkin's Lymphoma. Seminars in nuclear medicine. 2017;47:242-57.

[25] Elstrom R, Guan L, Baker G, Nakhoda K, Vergilio JA, Zhuang H, et al. Utility of FDG-PET scanning in lymphoma by WHO classification. Blood. 2003;101:3875-6.

[26] Caraway NP. Evolving role of FNA biopsy in diagnosing lymphoma: past, present, and future. Cancer cytopathology. 2015;123:389-93.

[27] Kung FH, Schwartz CL, Ferree CR, London WB, Ternberg JL, Behm FG, et al. POG 8625: a randomized trial comparing chemotherapy with chemoradiotherapy for children and adolescents with Stages I, IIA, IIIA1 Hodgkin Disease: a report from the Children's Oncology Group. Journal of pediatric hematology/oncology. 2006;28:362-8.

[28] Mauz-Korholz C, Metzger ML, Kelly KM, Schwartz CL, Castellanos ME, Dieckmann K, et al. Pediatric Hodgkin Lymphoma. Journal of clinical oncology : official journal of the American Society of Clinical Oncology. 2015;33:2975-85.

[29] Kahn JM, Ozuah NW, Dunleavy K, Henderson TO, Kelly K, LaCasce A. Adolescent and young adult lymphoma: collaborative efforts toward optimizing care and improving outcomes. Blood advances. 2017;1:1945-58.

[30] Simon JH, Paulino AC, Smith RB, Buatti JM. Prognostic factors in head and neck rhabdomyosarcoma. Head & neck. 2002;24:468-73.

[31] Miller RW, Young JL, Jr., Novakovic B. Childhood cancer. Cancer. 1995;75:395-405.

[32] Dasgupta R, Fuchs J, Rodeberg D. Rhabdomyosarcoma. Seminars in pediatric surgery. 2016;25:276-83.

[33] Dasgupta R, Rodeberg DA. Update on rhabdomyosarcoma. Seminars in pediatric surgery. 2012;21:68-78.

[34] Leaphart C, Rodeberg D. Pediatric surgical oncology: management of rhabdomyosarcoma. Surgical oncology. 2007;16:173-85.

[35] Pappo AS, Meza JL, Donaldson SS, Wharam MD, Wiener ES, Qualman SJ, et al. Treatment of localized nonorbital, nonparameningeal head and neck rhabdomyosarcoma: lessons learned from intergroup rhabdomyosarcoma studies III and IV. Journal of clinical oncology : official journal of the American Society of Clinical Oncology. 2003;21:638-45.

[36] Pappo AS, Shapiro DN, Crist WM, Maurer HM. Biology and therapy of pediatric rhabdomyosarcoma. Journal of clinical oncology : official journal of the American Society of Clinical Oncology. 1995;13:2123-39.

[37] Coffin CM, Davis JL, Borinstein SC. Syndrome-associated soft tissue tumours. Histopathology. 2014;64:68-87.

[38] Huh WW, Skapek SX. Childhood rhabdomyosarcoma: new insight on biology and treatment. Current oncology reports. 2010;12:402-10.

[39] Ognjanovic S, Linabery AM, Charbonneau B, Ross JA. Trends in childhood rhabdomyosarcoma incidence and survival in the United States, 1975-2005. Cancer. 2009;115:4218-26.

[40] Katal S, Gholamrezanezhad A, Kessler M, Olyaei M, Jadvar H. PET in the Diagnostic Management of Soft Tissue Sarcomas of Musculoskeletal Origin. PET clinics. 2018;13:609-21.

[41] Kumar R, Shandal V, Shamim SA, Halanaik D, Malhotra A. Clinical applications of PET and PET/CT in pediatric malignancies. Expert review of anticancer therapy. 2010;10:755-68.

[42] Mody RJ, Bui C, Hutchinson RJ, Yanik GA, Castle VP, Frey KA, et al. FDG PET imaging of childhood sarcomas. Pediatric blood & cancer. 2010;54:222-7.

[43] Tateishi U, Hosono A, Makimoto A, Nakamoto Y, Kaneta T, Fukuda H, et al. Comparative study of FDG PET/CT and conventional imaging in the staging of rhabdomyosarcoma. Annals of nuclear medicine. 2009;23:155-61.

[44] Rodeberg DA, Garcia-Henriquez N, Lyden ER, Davicioni E, Parham DM, Skapek SX, et al. Prognostic significance and tumor biology of regional lymph node disease in patients with rhabdomyosarcoma: a report from the Children's Oncology Group. Journal of clinical oncology : official journal of the American Society of Clinical Oncology. 2011;29:1304-11.

[45] Crist W, Gehan EA, Ragab AH, Dickman PS, Donaldson SS, Fryer C, et al. The Third Intergroup Rhabdomyosarcoma Study. Journal of clinical oncology : official journal of the American Society of Clinical Oncology. 1995;13:610-30.

[46] Crist WM, Anderson JR, Meza JL, Fryer C, Raney RB, Ruymann FB, et al. Intergroup rhabdomyosarcoma study-IV: results for patients with nonmetastatic disease. Journal of clinical oncology : official journal of the

American Society of Clinical Oncology. 2001;19:3091-102.

[47] Maurer HM, Beltangady M, Gehan EA, Crist W, Hammond D, Hays DM, et al. The Intergroup Rhabdomyosarcoma Study-I. A final report. Cancer. 1988;61:209-20.

[48] Maurer HM, Gehan EA, Beltangady M, Crist W, Dickman PS, Donaldson SS, et al. The Intergroup Rhabdomyosarcoma Study-II. Cancer. 1993;71:1904-22.

[49] Daya H, Chan HS, Sirkin W, Forte V. Pediatric rhabdomyosarcoma of the head and neck: is there a place for surgical management? Archives of otolaryngology--head & neck surgery. 2000;126:468-72.

[50] Walterhouse DO, Pappo AS, Baker KS, Parham DM, Anderson JR, Donaldson SS, et al. Rhabdomyosarcoma of the parotid region occurring in childhood and adolescence. A report from the Intergroup Rhabdomyosarcoma Study Group. Cancer. 2001;92:3135-46.

[51] Wiener ES. Head and neck rhabdomyosarcoma. Seminars in pediatric surgery. 1994;3:203-6.

[52] Raney B, Huh W, Hawkins D, Hayes-Jordan A, Million L, Rodeberg D, et al. Outcome of patients with localized orbital sarcoma who relapsed following treatment on Intergroup Rhabdomyosarcoma Study Group (IRSG) Protocols-III and -IV, 1984-1997: a report from the Children's Oncology Group. Pediatric blood & cancer. 2013;60:371-6.

[53] Hawkins DS, Anderson JR, Paidas CN, Wharam MD, Qualman SJ, Pappo AS, et al. Improved outcome for patients with middle ear rhabdomyosarcoma: a children's oncology group study. Journal of clinical oncology : official journal of the American Society of Clinical Oncology. 2001;19:3073-9.

[54] Reilly BK, Kim A, Pena MT, Dong TA, Rossi C, Murnick JG, et al. Rhabdomyosarcoma of the head and neck in children: review and update. International journal of pediatric otorhinolaryngology. 2015;79:1477-83.

[55] Hogan AR, Zhuge Y, Perez EA, Koniaris LG, Lew JI, Sola JE. Pediatric thyroid carcinoma: incidence and outcomes in 1753 patients. The Journal of surgical research. 2009;156:167-72.

[56] Shapiro NL, Bhattacharyya N. Population-based outcomes for pediatric thyroid carcinoma. The Laryngoscope. 2005;115:337-40.

[57] Niedziela M. Pathogenesis, diagnosis and management of thyroid nodules in children. Endocrine-related cancer. 2006;13:427-53.

[58] Dermody S, Walls A, Harley EH, Jr. Pediatric thyroid cancer: An update from the SEER database 2007-2012. International journal of pediatric otorhinolaryngology. 2016;89:121-6.

[59] La Quaglia MP, Black T, Holcomb GW, 3rd, Sklar C, Azizkhan RG, Haase GM, et al. Differentiated thyroid cancer: clinical characteristics, treatment, and outcome in patients under 21 years of age who present with distant metastases. A report from the Surgical Discipline Committee of the Children's Cancer Group. Journal of pediatric surgery. 2000;35:955-9; discussion 60.

[60] Astl J, Chovanec M, Lukes P, Katra R, Dvorakova M, Vlcek P, et al. Thyroid carcinoma surgery in children and adolescents - 15 years experience surgery of pediatric thyroid carcinoma. International journal of pediatric otorhinolaryngology. 2014;78:990-4.

[61] Diesen DL, Skinner MA. Pediatric thyroid cancer. Seminars in pediatric surgery. 2012;21:44-50.

[62] Spinelli C, Strambi S, Rossi L, Bakkar S, Massimino M, Ferrari A, et al. Surgical management of papillary thyroid carcinoma in childhood and adolescence: an Italian multicenter study on 250 patients. Journal of endocrinological investigation. 2016;39:1055-9.

[63] Acharya S, Sarafoglou K, LaQuaglia M, Lindsley S, Gerald W, Wollner N, et al. Thyroid neoplasms after therapeutic radiation for malignancies during childhood or adolescence. Cancer. 2003;97:2397-403.

[64] Constine LS, Tarbell N, Hudson MM, Schwartz C, Fisher SG, Muhs AG, et al. Subsequent malignancies in children treated for Hodgkin's disease: associations with gender and radiation dose. Int J Radiat Oncol Biol Phys. 2008;72:24-33.

[65] von der Weid NX. Adult life after surviving lymphoma in childhood. Supportive care in cancer : official journal of the Multinational Association of Supportive Care in Cancer. 2008;16:339-45.

[66] Buryk MA, Simons JP, Picarsic J, Monaco SE, Ozolek JA, Joyce J, et al. Can malignant thyroid nodules be distinguished from benign thyroid nodules in children and adolescents by clinical characteristics? A review of 89 pediatric patients with thyroid nodules. Thyroid : official journal of the American Thyroid Association. 2015;25:392-400.

[67] Koltin D, O'Gorman CS, Murphy A, Ngan B, Daneman A, Navarro OM, et al. Pediatric thyroid nodules: ultrasonographic characteristics and inter-observer variability in prediction of malignancy. Journal of pediatric endocrinology & metabolism : JPEM. 2016;29:789-94.

[68] Mussa A, De Andrea M, Motta M, Mormile A, Palestini N, Corrias A. Predictors of Malignancy in Children with Thyroid Nodules. The Journal of pediatrics. 2015;167:886-92.e1.

[69] Richman DM, Benson CB, Doubilet PM, Peters HE, Huang SA, Asch E, et al. Thyroid Nodules in Pediatric Patients: Sonographic Characteristics and Likelihood of Cancer. Radiology. 2018;288:591-9.

[70] Costante G, Meringolo D, Durante C, Bianchi D, Nocera M, Tumino S, et al. Predictive value of serum calcitonin levels for preoperative diagnosis of medullary thyroid carcinoma in a cohort of 5817 consecutive patients with thyroid nodules. The Journal of clinical endocrinology and metabolism. 2007;92:450-5.

[71] Francis GL, Waguespack SG, Bauer AJ, Angelos P, Benvenga S, Cerutti JM, et al. Management Guidelines for Children with Thyroid Nodules and Differentiated Thyroid Cancer. Thyroid : official journal of the American Thyroid Association. 2015;25:716-59.

[72] Nice T, Pasara S, Goldfarb M, Doski J, Goldin A, Gow KW, et al. Pediatric papillary thyroid cancer >1 cm: is total thyroidectomy necessary? Journal of pediatric surgery. 2015;50:1009-13.

[73] Bargren AE, Meyer-Rochow GY, Delbridge LW, Sidhu SB, Chen H. Outcomes of surgically managed pediatric thyroid cancer. The Journal of surgical research. 2009;156:70-3.

[74] Moley JF. Medullary thyroid carcinoma: management of lymph node metastases. Journal of the National Comprehensive Cancer Network : JNCCN. 2010;8:549-56.

[75] Wells SA, Jr., Pacini F, Robinson BG, Santoro M. Multiple endocrine

neoplasia type 2 and familial medullary thyroid carcinoma: an update. The Journal of clinical endocrinology and metabolism. 2013;98:3149-64.

[76] Mulligan LM, Marsh DJ, Robinson BG, Schuffenecker I, Zedenius J, Lips CJ, et al. Genotype-phenotype correlation in multiple endocrine neoplasia type 2: report of the International RET Mutation Consortium. Journal of internal medicine. 1995;238:343-6.

[77] Farndon JR, Leight GS, Dilley WG, Baylin SB, Smallridge RC, Harrison TS, et al. Familial medullary thyroid carcinoma without associated endocrinopathies: a distinct clinical entity. The British journal of surgery. 1986;73:278-81.

[78] Lallier M, St-Vil D, Giroux M, Huot C, Gaboury L, Oligny L, et al. Prophylactic thyroidectomy for medullary thyroid carcinoma in gene carriers of MEN2 syndrome. Journal of pediatric surgery. 1998;33:846-8.

[79] Moore SW, Appfelstaedt J, Zaahl MG. Familial medullary carcinoma prevention, risk evaluation, and RET in children of families with MEN2. Journal of pediatric surgery. 2007;42:326-32.

[80] Machens A, Niccoli-Sire P, Hoegel J, Frank-Raue K, van Vroonhoven TJ, Roeher HD, et al. Early malignant progression of hereditary medullary thyroid cancer. The New England journal of medicine. 2003;349:1517-25.

[81] Gomez IGC, Ponce Marco JL, Belda Ibanez T, Bosca Robledo A, Sebastian Pastor C, Navarro Milla R, et al. The optimal age for performing surgery on patients with MEN 2B syndrome. Oncology letters. 2011;2:929-30.

[82] Brandi ML, Gagel RF, Angeli A, Bilezikian JP, Beck-Peccoz P, Bordi C, et al. Guidelines for diagnosis and therapy of MEN type 1 and type 2. The Journal of clinical endocrinology and metabolism. 2001;86:5658-71.

[83] Spinelli C, Strambi S, Rossi L, Elisei R, Massimino M. Surgical Management of Medullary Thyroid Carcinoma in Pediatric Age. Current pediatric reviews. 2016;12:280-5.

[84] Albano D, Bertagna F, Panarotto MB, Giubbini R. Early and late adverse effects of radioiodine for pediatric differentiated thyroid cancer. Pediatric blood & cancer. 2017;64.

[85] Chow SM, Yau S, Lee SH, Leung WM, Law SC. Pregnancy outcome after diagnosis of differentiated thyroid carcinoma: no deleterious effect after radioactive iodine treatment. Int J Radiat Oncol Biol Phys. 2004;59:992-1000.

[86] Pawelczak M, David R, Franklin B, Kessler M, Lam L, Shah B. Outcomes of children and adolescents with well-differentiated thyroid carcinoma and pulmonary metastases following (1)(3)(1)I treatment: a systematic review. Thyroid : official journal of the American Thyroid Association. 2010;20:1095-101.

[87] Pao WJ, Hustu HO, Douglass EC, Beckford NS, Kun LE. Pediatric nasopharyngeal carcinoma: long term follow-up of 29 patients. Int J Radiat Oncol Biol Phys. 1989;17:299-305.

[88] Ayan I, Altun M. Nasopharyngeal carcinoma in children: retrospective review of 50 patients. Int J Radiat Oncol Biol Phys. 1996;35:485-92.

[89] Ozyar E, Selek U, Laskar S, Uzel O, Anacak Y, Ben-Arush M, et al. Treatment results of 165 pediatric patients with non-metastatic nasopharyngeal carcinoma: a Rare Cancer Network study. Radiotherapy and oncology : journal of the European Society for Therapeutic Radiology and Oncology. 2006;81:39-46.

[90] Mertens R, Granzen B, Lassay L, Bucsky P, Hundgen M, Stetter G, et al. Treatment of nasopharyngeal carcinoma in children and adolescents: definitive results of a multicenter study (NPC-91-GPOH). Cancer. 2005;104:1083-9.

[91] Ayan I, Kaytan E, Ayan N. Childhood nasopharyngeal carcinoma: from biology to treatment. The Lancet Oncology. 2003;4:13-21.

[92] Noorizan Y, Chew YK, Khir A, Brito-Mutunayagam S. Nasopharyngeal carcinoma: recognizing it early in children with otitis media with effusion. The Medical journal of Malaysia. 2008;63:261-2.

[93] Cvitkovic E, Bachouchi M, Armand JP. Nasopharyngeal carcinoma. Biology, natural history, and therapeutic implications. Hematology/oncology clinics of North America. 1991;5:821-38.

[94] Zubizarreta PA, D'Antonio G, Raslawski E, Gallo G, Preciado MV, Casak SJ, et al. Nasopharyngeal carcinoma in childhood and adolescence: a single-institution experience with combined therapy. Cancer. 2000;89:690-5.

[95] Toro C, Rinaldo A, Silver CE, Politi M, Ferlito A. Paraneoplastic syndromes in patients with nasopharyngeal cancer. Auris, nasus, larynx. 2009;36:513-20.

[96] Zhou GQ, Ren XY, Mao YP, Chen L, Sun Y, Liu LZ, et al. Prognostic implications of dynamic serum lactate dehydrogenase assessments in nasopharyngeal carcinoma patients treated with intensity-modulated radiotherapy. Scientific reports. 2016;6:22326.

[97] Zhang M, Wei S, Su L, Lv W, Hong J. Prognostic significance of pretreated serum lactate dehydrogenase level in nasopharyngeal carcinoma among Chinese population: A meta-analysis. Medicine. 2016;95:e4494.

[98] Mertens R, Granzen B, Lassay L, Gademann G, Hess CF, Heimann G. Nasopharyngeal carcinoma in childhood and adolescence: concept and preliminary results of the cooperative GPOH study NPC-91. Gesellschaft fur Padiatrische Onkologie und Hamatologie. Cancer. 1997;80:951-9.

[99] Ingersoll L, Woo SY, Donaldson S, Giesler J, Maor MH, Goffinet D, et al. Nasopharyngeal carcinoma in the young: a combined M.D. Anderson and Stanford experience. Int J Radiat Oncol Biol Phys. 1990;19:881-7.

[100] Langendijk JA, Leemans CR, Buter J, Berkhof J, Slotman BJ. The additional value of chemotherapy to radiotherapy in locally advanced nasopharyngeal carcinoma: a meta-analysis of the published literature. Journal of clinical oncology : official journal of the American Society of Clinical Oncology. 2004;22:4604-12.

[101] Nikitovic M, Popovic-Vukovic M, Stanic D, Bokun J, Paripovic L, Ilic V, et al. Treatment outcome of childhood nasopharyngeal carcinoma: A single institution experience. International journal of pediatric otorhinolaryngology. 2018;113:168-72.

[102] Cooper JS, Lee H, Torrey M, Hochster H. Improved outcome secondary to concurrent chemoradiotherapy for advanced carcinoma of the nasopharynx: preliminary corroboration of the intergroup experience. Int J Radiat Oncol Biol Phys. 2000;47:861-6.

[103] Chua MLK, Wee JTS, Hui EP, Chan ATC. Nasopharyngeal carcinoma. Lancet (London, England). 2016;387:1012-24.

[104] Casanova M, Bisogno G, Gandola L, Cecchetto G, Di Cataldo A,

Basso E, et al. A prospective protocol for nasopharyngeal carcinoma in children and adolescents: the Italian Rare Tumors in Pediatric Age (TREP) project. Cancer. 2012;118:2718-25.

[105] Wolden SL, Steinherz PG, Kraus DH, Zelefsky MJ, Pfister DG, Wollner N. Improved long-term survival with combined modality therapy for pediatric nasopharynx cancer. Int J Radiat Oncol Biol Phys. 2000;46:859-64.

[106] Jenkin RD, Anderson JR, Jereb B, Thompson JC, Pyesmany A, Wara WM, et al. Nasopharyngeal carcinoma--a retrospective review of patients less than thirty years of age: a report of Children's Cancer Study Group. Cancer. 1981;47:360-6.

[107] Serin M, Erkal HS, Elhan AH, Cakmak A. Nasopharyngeal carcinoma in childhood and adolescence. Medical and pediatric oncology. 1998;31:498-505.

[108] Cheuk DK, Billups CA, Martin MG, Roland CR, Ribeiro RC, Krasin MJ, et al. Prognostic factors and long-term outcomes of childhood nasopharyngeal carcinoma. Cancer. 2011;117:197-206.

[109] Vokes EE, Liebowitz DN, Weichselbaum RR. Nasopharyngeal carcinoma. Lancet (London, England). 1997;350:1087-91.

[110] Uzel O, Yoruk SO, Sahinler I, Turkan S, Okkan S. Nasopharyngeal carcinoma in childhood: long-term results of 32 patients. Radiotherapy and oncology : journal of the European Society for Therapeutic Radiology and Oncology. 2001;58:137-41.

[111] Yoshida EJ, Garcia J, Eisele DW, Chen AM. Salivary gland malignancies in children. International journal of pediatric otorhinolaryngology. 2014;78:174-8.

[112] Aro K, Leivo I, Makitie A. Management of salivary gland malignancies in the pediatric population. Current opinion in otolaryngology & head and neck surgery. 2014;22:116-20.

[113] Krolls SO, Trodahl JN, Boyers RC. Salivary gland lesions in children. A survey of 430 cases. Cancer. 1972;30:459-69.

[114] Fang QG, Shi S, Li ZN, Zhang X, Liu FY, Sun CF. Epithelial salivary gland tumors in children: a twenty-five-year experience of 122 patients. International journal of pediatric otorhinolaryngology. 2013;77:1252-4.

[115] Cockerill CC, Gross BC, Contag S, Rein S, Moore EJ, Olsen KD, et al. Pediatric malignant salivary gland tumors: 60 year follow up. International journal of pediatric otorhinolaryngology. 2016;88:1-6.

[116] Ribeiro Kde C, Kowalski LP, Saba LM, de Camargo B. Epithelial salivary glands neoplasms in children and adolescents: a forty-four-year experience. Medical and pediatric oncology. 2002;39:594-600.

[117] Sultan I, Rodriguez-Galindo C, Al-Sharabati S, Guzzo M, Casanova M, Ferrari A. Salivary gland carcinomas in children and adolescents: a population-based study, with comparison to adult cases. Head & neck. 2011;33:1476-81.

[118] Callender DL, Frankenthaler RA, Luna MA, Lee SS, Goepfert H. Salivary gland neoplasms in children. Archives of otolaryngology--head & neck surgery. 1992;118:472-6.

[119] Kessler A, Handler SD. Salivary gland neoplasms in children: a 10-year survey at the Children's Hospital of Philadelphia. International journal of pediatric otorhinolaryngology. 1994;29:195-202.

[120] Verma J, Teh BS, Paulino AC. Characteristics and outcome of radiation and chemotherapy-related mucoepidermoid carcinoma of the salivary glands. Pediatric blood & cancer. 2011;57:1137-41.

[121] Vedrine PO, Coffinet L, Temam S, Montagne K, Lapeyre M, Oberlin O, et al. Mucoepidermoid carcinoma of salivary glands in the pediatric age group: 18 clinical cases, including 11 second malignant neoplasms. Head & neck. 2006;28:827-33.

[122] DeLaat CA, Lampkin BC. Long-term survivors of childhood cancer: evaluation and identification of sequelae of treatment. CA: a cancer journal for clinicians. 1992;42:263-82.

[123] Preston-Martin S, Thomas DC, White SC, Cohen D. Prior exposure to medical and dental x-rays related to tumors of the parotid gland. Journal of the National Cancer Institute. 1988;80:943-9.

[124] Land CE, Saku T, Hayashi Y, Takahara O, Matsuura H, Tokuoka S, et al. Incidence of salivary gland tumors among atomic bomb survivors, 1950-1987. Evaluation of radiation-related risk. Radiation research. 1996;146:28-36.

[125] Guzzo M, Locati LD, Prott FJ, Gatta G, McGurk M, Licitra *L. major* and minor salivary gland tumors. Critical reviews in oncology/hematology. 2010;74:134-48.

[126] Orvidas LJ, Kasperbauer JL, Lewis JE, Olsen KD, Lesnick TG. Pediatric parotid masses. Archives of otolaryngology--head & neck surgery. 2000;126:177-84.

[127] Lee DH, Yoon TM, Lee JK, Lim SC. Clinical utility of fine needle aspiration cytology in pediatric parotid tumors. International journal of pediatric otorhinolaryngology. 2013;77:1272-5.

[128] Koyuncu M, Sesen T, Akan H, Ismailoglu AA, Tanyeri Y, Tekat A, et al. Comparison of computed tomography and magnetic resonance imaging in the diagnosis of parotid tumors. Otolaryngology--head and neck surgery : official journal of American Academy of Otolaryngology-Head and Neck Surgery. 2003;129:726-32.

[129] Eveson JW. Salivary tumours. Periodontology 2000. 2011;57:150-9.

[130] Shikhani AH, Johns ME. Tumors of the major salivary glands in children. Head & neck surgery. 1988;10:257-63.

[131] Andry G, Hamoir M, Locati LD, Licitra L, Langendijk JA. Management of salivary gland tumors. Expert review of anticancer therapy. 2012;12:1161-8.

[132] Rahbar R, Grimmer JF, Vargas SO, Robson CD, Mack JW, Perez-Atayde AR, et al. Mucoepidermoid carcinoma of the parotid gland in children: A 10-year experience. Archives of otolaryngology--head & neck surgery. 2006;132:375-80.

[133] Thariat J, Vedrine PO, Temam S, Ali AM, Orbach D, Odin G, et al. The role of radiation therapy in pediatric mucoepidermoid carcinomas of the salivary glands. The Journal of pediatrics. 2013;162:839-43.

[134] Brady JS, Chung SY, Marchiano E, Eloy JA, Baredes S, Park RCW. Pediatric head and neck bone sarcomas: An analysis of 204 cases. International journal of pediatric otorhinolaryngology. 2017;100:71-6.

[135] Trosman SJ, Krakovitz PR. Pediatric maxillary and mandibular tumors. Otolaryngologic clinics of North America. 2015;48:101-19.

[136] Huh WW, Fitzgerald N, Mahajan A, Sturgis EM, Beverly Raney R, Anderson PM. Pediatric sarcomas and related tumors of the head

and neck. Cancer treatment reviews. 2011;37:431-9.

[137] Peng KA, Grogan T, Wang MB. Head and neck sarcomas: analysis of the SEER database. Otolaryngology--head and neck surgery : official journal of American Academy of Otolaryngology-Head and Neck Surgery. 2014;151:627-33.

[138] Daw NC, Mahmoud HH, Meyer WH, Jenkins JJ, Kaste SC, Poquette CA, et al. Bone sarcomas of the head and neck in children: the St Jude Children's Research Hospital experience. Cancer. 2000;88:2172-80.

[139] Ottaviani G, Jaffe N. The epidemiology of osteosarcoma. Cancer treatment and research. 2009;152:3-13.

[140] Alam K, Khan R, Jain A, Maheshwari V, Agrawal S, Chana RS, et al. The value of fine-needle aspiration cytology in the evaluation of pediatric head and neck tumors. International journal of pediatric otorhinolaryngology. 2009;73:923-7.

[141] Gibson SE, Prayson RA. Primary skull lesions in the pediatric population: a 25-year experience. Archives of pathology & laboratory medicine. 2007;131:761-6.

[142] Patel SG, Meyers P, Huvos AG, Wolden S, Singh B, Shaha AR, et al. Improved outcomes in patients with osteogenic sarcoma of the head and neck. Cancer. 2002;95:1495-503.

[143] Gadwal SR, Gannon FH, Fanburg-Smith JC, Becoskie EM, Thompson LD. Primary osteosarcoma of the head and neck in pediatric patients: a clinicopathologic study of 22 cases with a review of the literature. Cancer. 2001;91:598-605.

[144] Fernandes R, Nikitakis NG, Pazoki A, Ord RA. Osteogenic sarcoma of the jaw: a 10-year experience. Journal of oral and maxillofacial surgery : official journal of the American Association of Oral and Maxillofacial Surgeons. 2007;65:1286-91.

[145] Allison DC, Carney SC, Ahlmann ER, Hendifar A, Chawla S, Fedenko A, et al. A meta-analysis of osteosarcoma outcomes in the modern medical era. Sarcoma. 2012;2012:704872.

[146] Sun Y, Liu X, Pan S, Deng C, Li X, Guo Q. Analysis of imaging characteristics of primary malignant bone tumors in children. Oncology letters. 2017;14:5801-10.

[147] Costelloe CM, Madewell JE. Radiography in the initial diagnosis of primary bone tumors. AJR American journal of roentgenology. 2013;200:3-7.

[148] Kaste SC. Imaging pediatric bone sarcomas. Radiologic clinics of North America. 2011;49:749-65, vi-vii.

[149] Klein MJ, Siegal GP. Osteosarcoma: anatomic and histologic variants. American journal of clinical pathology. 2006;125:555-81.

[150] Chui MH, Kandel RA, Wong M, Griffin AM, Bell RS, Blackstein ME, et al. Histopathologic Features of Prognostic Significance in High-Grade Osteosarcoma. Archives of pathology & laboratory medicine. 2016.

[151] Nie Z, Peng H. Osteosarcoma in patients below 25 years of age: An observational study of incidence, metastasis, treatment and outcomes. Oncology letters. 2018;16:6502-14.

[152] Kaste SC, Fuller CE, Saharia A, Neel MD, Rao BN, Daw NC. Pediatric surface osteosarcoma: clinical, pathologic, and radiologic features. Pediatric blood & cancer. 2006;47:152-62.

[153] Price CH, Zhuber K, Salzer-Kuntschik M, Salzer M,

Willert HG, Immenkamp M, et al. Osteosarcoma in children. A study of 125 cases. The Journal of bone and joint surgery British volume. 1975;57:341-5.

[154] Smeele LE, van der Wal JE, van Diest PJ, van der Waal I, Snow GB. Radical surgical treatment in craniofacial osteosarcoma gives excellent survival. A retrospective cohort study of 14 patients. European journal of cancer Part B, Oral oncology. 1994;30b:374-6.

[155] Huh WW, Holsinger FC, Levy A, Palla FS, Anderson PM. Osteosarcoma of the jaw in children and young adults. Head & neck. 2012;34:981-4.

[156] Chen Y, Shen Q, Gokavarapu S, Lin C, Yahiya, Cao W, et al. Osteosarcoma of head and neck: A retrospective study on prognostic factors from a single institute database. Oral oncology. 2016;58:1-7.

[157] Guadagnolo BA, Zagars GK, Raymond AK, Benjamin RS, Sturgis EM. Osteosarcoma of the jaw/craniofacial region: outcomes after multimodality treatment. Cancer. 2009;115:3262-70.

Section 2

Head and Neck Reconstruction

Chapter 3

Reconstruction of Pharyngeal Defects

Takako Yabe and Bruce Ashford

Abstract

The management of pharyngeal defects is one of the most challenging tasks for reconstructive surgeons. The reconstructive method is driven by the amount of tissue loss as well as patient-related factors. Since the advent of organ preservation strategies in the 1990s as described by the Department of Veterans Affairs Laryngeal Cancer Study, salvage surgery has become a common pharyngeal procedure to obtain local control when nonsurgical treatment fails. This chapter is divided into preoperative, intraoperative, and postoperative phases of patient management. Each section will focus on particular aspects of management that are essential to achieve the best therapeutic outcome for patients who need pharyngeal reconstruction.

Keywords: head and neck reconstruction, pharynx, hypopharyngectomy, pedicled flaps, microvascular free flaps

1. Introduction

The pharynx is a muscular column that begins posterior to the nasal cavity, descends inferiorly behind the oral cavity before merging with the larynx and the oesophagus. It is subdivided into nasopharynx, oropharynx and hypopharynx (laryngopharynx) based on their anterior relations. Its primary functions are both digestive and respiratory where it creates the passage for air, solids, and liquids from the nose and mouth. Hypopharynx guides food into the oesophagus and pharyngeal muscles further support deglutition and speech.

Oncologic management of the pharynx presents complex challenges for both ablative and reconstructive surgeons. The move away from surgical management of both laryngeal (VA study) and pharyngeal malignancy has meant that many patients eventually presenting to surgery do so in a salvage setting. With the advent of transoral robotic surgery (TORS), a reframing of the role of surgery in the management of pharyngeal malignancy is underway. The results of Eastern Cooperative Oncology Group (ECOG-ACRIN 3311) may prescribe an increased role for TORS and impact on reconstructive strategies. ECOG-ACRIN 3311 examines reduced postoperative therapy in patients with "intermediate risk" p16+ oropharynx cancer (OPC) undergoing primary transoral surgical management. E3311 was a phase II randomised clinical trial of transoral surgery followed by low- or standard-dose, risk-adjusted post-operative radiotherapy with stage III-IVa (AJCC 7th edition) HPV associated oropharyngeal cancer (OPC). In this chapter, we will outline the range of requirements for pharyngeal reconstruction, and to outline the options for the surgeon managing pharyngeal defect reconstruction.

The 5-year survival rate of pharyngeal squamous cell carcinoma (SCC) depends on tumour stage and human papillomavirus (HPV) status. Up to 60% of patients die within three years [1]. However, beyond oncologic outcomes, functionality and quality of survival is an important determinant of therapy. The physiologic cost of surgery needs to be balanced against the well known long term effects of non-surgical therapies. The role of the reconstructive surgeon is to manage short term perioperative problems and long term functional outcomes to achieve the optimal quality of life result for the patient [2].

The practice changing Department of Veterans Affairs Laryngeal Cancer Study was a prospective, randomised study in patients with previously untreated advanced (stage III or IV) laryngeal squamous carcinoma. This study compared the results of induction chemotherapy followed by definitive radiation therapy with those of conventional laryngectomy and postoperative radiation [3]. A significant finding of the study was that chemoradiation successfully preserved the larynx in 64% of the patients. They achieved this result with a 2-year survival rate equivalent to that of conventional laryngectomy and postoperative radiation therapy [3]. The Intergroup Radiation Therapy Oncology Group 91–11 (RTOG-91-11) study evaluated the contribution of chemotherapy added to radiation therapy for larynx preservation. It also documented that concurrent chemoradiotherapy for the treatment of advanced laryngeal carcinoma conferred the highest rate of organ preservation at 84% [4]. These landmark trials have effectively relegated the role of total laryngectomy to those cases where there is no organ function to preserve or are in the salvage setting with extra-laryngeal spread [5].

The extent of defect determines the extent of reconstruction required. For small pharyngeal defects, primary closure or healing by secondary intention with the acceptance of some distortion of the local pharyngeal contour might be acceptable in the non-salvage setting. Post radiation granulation or primary repair, regardless of the defect size, is an unpredictable clinical scenario which should be avoided. Rates of pharyngocutaneous fistula (PCF) are related to the size and complexity of the defect and prior (chemo)radiation. The incidence of PCF range from 9–23% depending on the clinical context [6]. It is the avoidance of PCF which mandates a nuanced approach to the management of the post-ablation pharynx and that is a primary determinant of early post-treatment quality of life. Reconstruction of pharyngeal defects with free tissue transfer or well vascularised regional tissue [7] is considered the preferred choice in the salvage setting [8]. Chemotherapy is known to affect the function of neutrophil, macrophage, as well as B-cell and T-cell functions, resulting in impaired cellular and humoral immunity [9]. Wound healing potential is further compromised by radiation-induced obliterative endarteritis and fibrosis [10]. Salvage surgery often necessitates a broad field extirpation of the neck and upper mediastinal tissues that results in bilateral carotid artery exposure. Deficient wound healing caused by both chemotherapy and radiotherapy predisposes this patient population to development of pharyngocutaneous salivary fistula and life-threatening vessel rupture from salivary contamination and sepsis [6].

The recent history of head and neck reconstructive surgery can be traced back to the early twentieth century with axial patterned island flaps, split-thickness skin grafts, and regional flaps [11]. Flaps generally refer to tissue reconstruction with an intact blood supply, whereas grafts imply a non-vascularised transfer of tissue. Microvascular free tissue transfers (flaps) are further differentiated from regional flaps that their vascular supply is temporarily disconnected from the systemic circulation to be transplanted to a recipient site. Free flap surgery gained popularity in the latter half of the twentieth century [12].

2. Pre-operative considerations: goals and planning

All forms of treatment for these pharyngeal/pharygolaryngeal malignancies carry considerable toxicity, particularly to deglutition [13, 14]. Surgery, which is increasingly used to salvage failures of organ-preservation therapy [15], has considerable morbidity and mortality [16, 17] more so than for any other type of head and neck cancer [18]. The complexity of care in the salvage setting is difficult to overstate.

Primary goals of reconstruction of pharyngeal defects are maintenance of integrity, restoration of function and form, minimising morbidity, and improving quality of life [19]. The reconstruction needs to be able to withstand adjuvant radiotherapy but be compliant enough to restore a range of three-dimensional defects [20].

The gold standard of reconstruction should be a one-stage procedure with the lowest morbidity, a short hospital stay, early recovery of swallowing, and the restoration of a socially acceptable appearance [2]. Given the aim of getting the patient to adjuvant therapy, achieving the seal of the pharynx to allow for the restoration of enteral feeding and avoidance of neck sepsis is crucial [21]. Precise preoperative planning, including thorough comorbidity evaluations, is mandatory in these patients. Preoperative nutritional assessment and optimisation and the normalisation of other systemic diseases, including particularly hypothyroidism are essential before any effort at pharyngeal reconstruction.

The reconstructive ladder describes an increasing complexity of options: healing by secondary intention, primary closure, grafts, local flaps, regional flaps then distant flaps [19]. The simplest surgical option may not necessarily be the best surgical option because it does not take into consideration the goals of reconstruction [22].

In the situations where all of the reconstructive goals cannot be satisfied, they should be prioritised in the following order as mentioned below [19];

1. Maintenance of the integrity of head and neck tissues and aerodigestive tract with isolation of the intracranial content.

2. Restoration of the form including facial contour, consistency, and dimension.

3. Minimisation of anaesthesia exposure, complications, and morbidity.

4. Improvements to the quality of life.

The seven principles of pharyngeal reconstruction are as follows [23];

1. Single-stage reconstruction

2. Restoration of deglutition

3. Restoration of speech

4. Toleration of radiotherapy

5. Successful reconstruction in a heavily irradiated field

6. Minimal morbidity at the donor site

7. Minimal morbidity at the reconstruction site

Reconstructive options should be explored and discussed during the planning phase before ablative surgery based on the following principles [19];

1. Surgical defect

2. Anatomy

3. Surgeon expertise

4. Surgical facility

5. Reconstructive goals

6. Patient factors (i.e. comorbidities, body habitus, cancer prognosis, history of radiation and surgery, family support, and personal wishes)

Within reason, and subject to unforeseen intraoperative requirements, the reconstructive plan should be well understood by both the ablative and reconstructive teams. The ablative surgeon needs to appreciate the need for vessel preservation (in the event of free flap for reconstruction) and also needs to communicate any changes to the plan so that the reconstructive team can pre-empt modifications that might be required. The surgical management and reconstruction of the vessel depleted neck are of a particular challenge, and this problem should have been at least known preoperatively [24].

3. Intra-operative considerations

3.1 Pharyngeal defect

The extent of pharyngeal defect after resection can range from a small tonsillar or sidewall defect to a circumferential defect resulting from laryngopharyngectomy. Smaller defects in the primary setting can be managed by secondary intention without any sophisticated reconstruction. Larger defects or those in the post-radiation setting are more likely to benefit from active efforts to re-establish the pharynx.

Defect type can be classified according to the amount of residual mucosa [25].

1. Defects not requiring closure

2. Defects with sufficient pharyngeal mucosa to close primarily

3. Defects where a strip of pharyngeal mucosa remains but is insufficient to close on itself

4. Complete circumferential defects where a 360-degree segment of pharyngeal mucosa is lacking

Hui et al. demonstrated that primary closure can be achieved with acceptable swallowing outcomes with a minimum of 1.5 cm of relaxed or 2.5 cm of stretched pharyngeal mucosa remaining [26]. In circumstances where there is sufficient mucosa to close a pharyngeal defect primarily, the current evidence generally favours onlay vascularised tissue over the suture line to reduce the rates of fistulation [10, 27].

A circumferential defect with the reconstruction of a neopharynx would, in most cases, be best managed with free tissue transfer, either as a "tubed" anterolateral thigh or radial forearm free flap or using some component of the alimentary tract such as the stomach or small bowel (**Figure 1**) [25].

3.2 Technical considerations

In a recent review on managing pharyngeal defects, Ragbir et al. indicated that pharyngeal defects with more than 3.5 cm of residual pharyngeal mucosa may be closed primarily, defects with less than 3.5 cm of residual pharyngeal mucosal width require interpositioning replacement with imported tissue, and circumferential pharyngeal defects require circumferential reconstruction.

Primary closure of pharyngeal defects can be performed in vertical, horizontal, or T shaped orientations. The ideal technique for closure and the resultant fistula rates have been intensely debated. Pioneering work by Su and Chian [28] advocated placement of the T-shaped suture line. Cho et al. [29] suggested a modification to the flap design by overlapping the vertical suture line with de-epithelialised skin and using a two-layered closure with triangular flaps at the distal anastomotic site. Although no consensus has been reached, it is important to remember the principles of closure; the approximation needs to be watertight with just adequate approximation to avoid compromising the vascularity of the suture line [30]. As with all tissue closures, tension should be avoided.

Where primary closure cannot be achieved safely, or in cases where primary closure has been possible in the salvage/post radiotherapy context, either coverage or augmentation of the closure with either a regional flap or a free tissue transfer may be necessary.

3.3 Flap choices

Most soft tissue flaps are designed to be 10 to 20% larger than the defect itself to accommodate for tissue shrinkage [19]. They can be pedicled or microvascular free

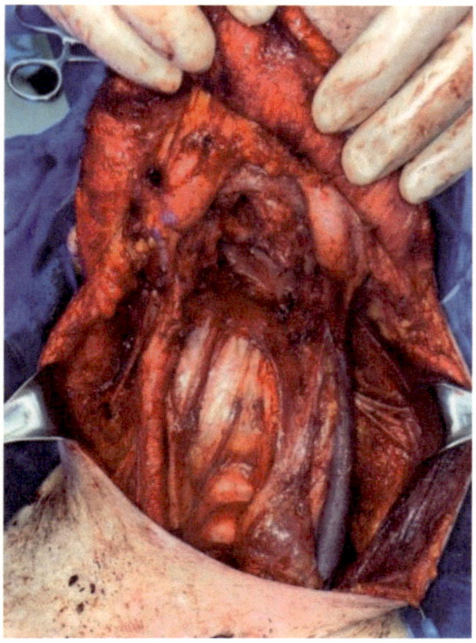

Figure 1.
Defect following salvage total pharyngolaryngectomy.

flaps depending on the nativity of their blood supply. Their advantages and disadvantages are discussed below.

3.3.1 Regional pedicle flap options

3.3.1.1 Pectoralis major myocutaneous flap

The pectoralis major (PM) flap was first described by Ariyan [31] in 1979. In the setting of pharyngeal defects, it can be grafted to a defect with or without a cutaneous component. Inset of an area of skin into a pharyngeal defect allows for a more robust seal to be achieved early. Without skin, the muscle flap can be used to seal a defect or to onlay over a primary pharyngeal closure. Using the PM pedicled flap as an onlay flap has been shown to decrease the rate of pharyngocutaneous fistula when compared to primary closure alone [32].

With a circumferential pharyngeal defect, the PM flap can be sutured directly to the prevertebral fascia or with a split-thickness skin graft relining the prevertebral fascia [33]. More commonly, the PM flap is used as a patch repair to reconstruct the anterior pharyngeal wall in cases where only the posterior wall remains [25].

Advantages include a relative ease of harvest and reduced operating time when compared to free tissue transfer. Moreover, the PM flap is a robust and reliable option that obviates the need for microsurgical anastomosis, which is particularly relevant in a vessel-depleted neck. The disadvantage of such a bulky flap is that it can create tension on the tongue which may limit tongue mobility, impairing speech, articulation and swallowing function. Even if the muscle is denervated, the relative bulkiness of the muscle often persists and this can also impede tracheo-esophageal speech by impairing the vibratory quality of the neopharynx [25]. Voice outcomes after PM flap reconstruction of the pharynx are shown to be inferior to those of primary closure alone [34].

Donor site morbidities, including shoulder and arm dysfunction as well as chest wall contour deformity are significant and debilitating. The muscular bulk of the flap can also distort the stoma, making the use of a voice prosthesis more challenging [35].

The PM pedicled flap is usually limited to the medically comorbid patient who would not otherwise tolerate the prolonged operating time under general anaesthesia required for a free flap. It is often utilised as a back-up flap in circumstances where wound breakdown compromises any initial pharyngeal reconstruction [25].

3.3.1.2 Supraclavicular artery island flap (SCAIF)

The SCAIF is a pedicled fasciocutaneous flap based on the supraclavicular artery and vein. These vessels arise from the transverse cervical vessels and this flap can be used for a multitude of head and neck reconstructions where a thin and pliable replacement is indicated [36]. Up to 20% of patients will not have the branch of the transverse cervical artery (TCA) [37] and preoperative audible doppler will allow for assessment of this vessel as it runs over the lateral clavicle into the deltoid region. Emerick et al. reported their experience using the SCAIF in reconstruction following total laryngectomy [35]. A benefit of the SCAIF is its ability to reconstruct the anterior neck skin, which may be necessary in the setting of salvage laryngectomy [35].

3.3.1.3 Internal mammary artery perforator flap (IMAP)

The IMAP is supplied by the first 3 or 4 branches of the internal mammary artery. It is raised in a subfascial plane to within 2–3 cm of the sternal margin. The flap is raised as an island to allow for rotation on a relatively short pedicle. Iyer et al.

suggested that it is a reliable and suitable option for lower anterior neck defect [38] including for revision of tracheostomes.

3.3.1.4 Thoracoacrominal artery perforator flap (TAAP)

The thoracoacrominal artery perforator (TAAP) flap is a local alternative solution for reconstruction of complex circumferential hypopharyngeal defects when free tissue transfer is contraindicated or neck vessels are depleted [39]. It can be harvested as a chimeric flap including both muscle and skin components to cover defects in pharynx as well as skin.

3.3.2 Free tissue transfer options

Free flaps can serve to

a. reinforce a primary closure (particularly in the post-radiation salvage setting),

b. as a patch or interposition for lost circumference or

c. as a "tubed" reconstruction in cases where circumferential pharyngeal reconstruction is required.

The introduction of a free flap harvested from outside the irradiated field helps improve vascularity in the wound bed, may aid with healing, and decrease the risk of wound complications. Subsequently, including a free flap as an onlay graft may also help even in situations where primary closure of the pharynx is otherwise possible [25]. A meta-analysis on risk factors by Sayle and Grant concluded that a flap-reinforced closure is warranted in the salvage setting and would be of the most significant benefit where patients had undergone concurrent chemoradiotherapy [40]. Significant reduction of the PCF rate was demonstrated by Higgins et al. when the temporoparietal fascia was used an onlay flap [41]. Fung et al. introduced the term "pharyngeal interposition graft" (PIG), which consist of fascia-only free flaps to improve tissue vascularity in salvage laryngectomy [10]. Paleri et al. demonstrated that the incorporation of vascularised flaps, as either a patch repair or as a PIG, reduced the rate of pharyngocutaneous fistula by one-third [42].

Free tissue transfer options for pharyngeal reconstruction include.

3.3.2.1 Radial forearm free flap

The radial forearm free flap (RFFF) is easy to harvest, has a long pedicle with excellent vessel calibre, and is made up of a thin, pliable skin paddle of variable size and form that allow a great deal of latitude in pharyngeal reconstruction [43]. Its long pedicle provides an option for vascular anastomosis to be performed on the contralateral neck.

One of the major advantages of this is that its inherently thin and pliable skin paddle matches the thickness of the pharyngoesophageal wall [43]. If there is sufficient mucosa to close the pharynx primarily, the RFFF can be harvested without a skin paddle as a fascia-only flap to reinforce the pharyngeal suture line.

3.3.2.2 Anterolateral thigh free flap

The anterolateral thigh free flap (ALT) can be used as an onlay, a patch, or a tubed flap. It has more considerable vascular variability when compared to the RFFF. Its thickness also varies significantly depending on a patient's body habitus. The excess adipose tissue can be removed to within 2 cm of the perforating vessel to limit the flap thickness [44]. The ALT can be raised as a chimeric flap with muscle (usually vastus lateralis). The muscle can serve to provide coverage of the great vessels in the case of concurrent radical neck dissections, to fill in neck contour defects, or as a vascularised bed to facilitate skin grafting for the external neck. A distal or a second skin paddle can be brought out to external skin and utilised as a monitoring paddle [45].

The main favourable characteristics of the ALT flap include reliable anatomy, long vascular pedicle, low donor-site morbidity, feasibility as a chimeric flap, and the possibility of an in-OR 2-team approach [46]. The ALT flap can provide up to 40 cm of length for oesophageal reconstruction, especially when folded in a conical fashion [47]. The donor site is closed primarily and typically, the only lasting sequelae include a vertically oriented scar along the thigh and thigh numbness (**Figures 2** and **3**).

3.3.2.3 Gastro-omental free flap

The gastro-omental flap was first described by Baudet [48] for use in 1979. It is typically raised via laparotomy although it can be harvested laparoscopically [49]. The flap provides a tubed segment of the greater curve of the stomach which is nourished by the right gastroepiploic artery and vein, which also supply an apron of omentum. The advantage of the gastro-omental flap is its unique wound-healing properties provided by the rich omental source of fibroblasts and other progenitor cells. The omentum also serves as a malleable vascularised layer over the microvascular anastomoses and protects the great vessels from contamination by salivary egress [50]. Fibrous adhesions form within 3 hours of flap inset, leading to rapid ingrowth of fibroblasts and capillaries, which provide a nutrient-rich bed ideally suited to facilitate healing in contaminated or chemoirradiated wounds [51].

Unlike the body of the stomach, the gastric antrum is sparsely populated by gastric parietal cells,. This theoretically avoids acid-secretion from the transferred tissues (**Figures 4** and 5) [50].

3.3.2.4 Jejunal free flap

The jejunal flap provides a hollow viscus which can replace a circumferential pharyngeal defect. It has a relatively shorter pedicle than the other free flaps herein

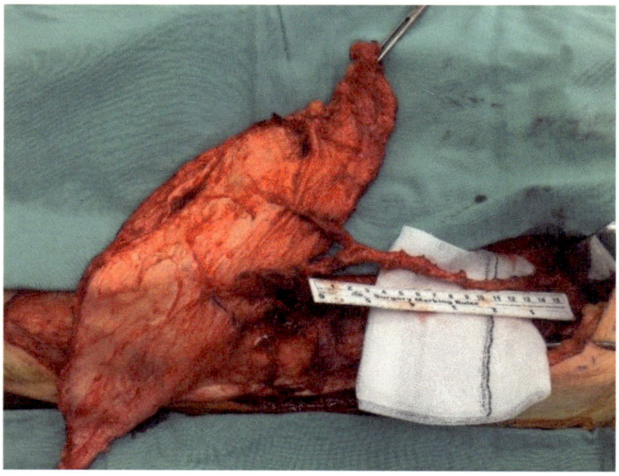

Figure 2.
ALT flap with pedicle.

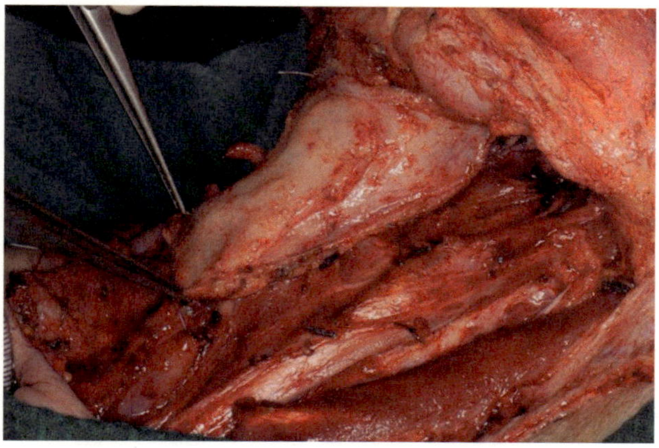

Figure 3.
Tubed ALT flap inset.

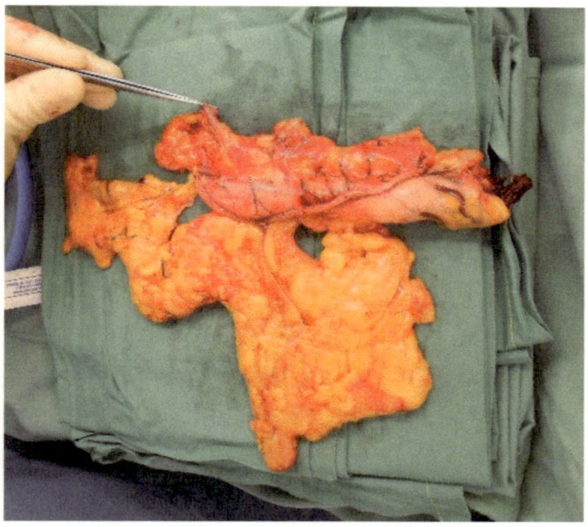

Figure 4.
Gastro-omental free flap.

described. A perioperative mortality rate was 3.8% in a series of 368 patients who had jejunal free flap for circumferential laryngopharyngectomy defects [52]. The potential morbidity of abdominal surgery such as postoperative ileus, wound infection, bowel obstruction, superior mesenteric syndrome, intra-abdominal bleeding, and delayed enteric feeding are significant complications in an already medically compromised population [53]. The jejunal flap is less tolerant of ischaemia and has a shorter pedicle than other flaps such as the ALT or gastro-omental flaps. The re-vascularised jejunal flap does not seem to withstand high doses radiotherapy [54]. Small bowel peristalsis generated by myenteric plexus does not seem to add any benefit to the pharyngeal phase of swallowing, as jejunal peristalsis does not coordinate with the rest of the upper digestive tract [25].

3.3.2.5 Temporoparietal fascial free flap

Temporoparietal fascial free flap (TPFF) is thin and pliable and can be used as a PIG to reinforce pharyngeal closures after salvage laryngectomy. Higgins et al. [41] demonstrated comparable wound outcomes to the pectoralis major myofascial flap without the associated shoulder and arm dysfunction. This flap has minimal donor site morbidity other than a 25% rate of local alopecia. The pedicle is short and with small calibre.

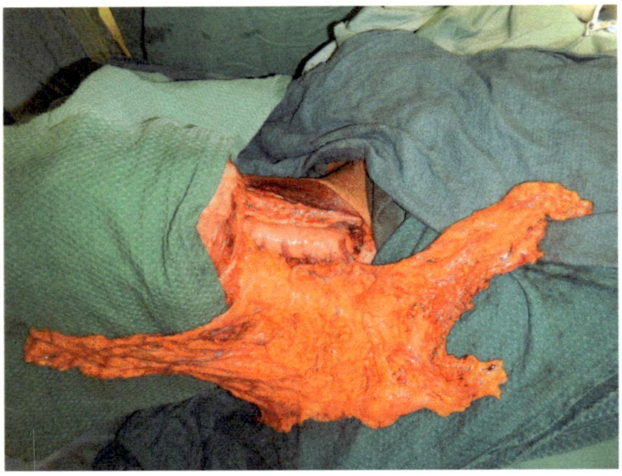

Figure 5.
Gastro-omental flap inset.

It is still possible to undertake a two-team approach if harvest commences after ipsilateral dissection is complete [41]. The use of the TPFF as an overlay technique is a useful adjunct for salvage laryngectomy cases where the defect is primarily closed. The reinforcement of the pharyngeal suture line has been shown to diminish the rate of PCF compared to historical controls with reduced donor-site morbidity and reduced length of hospitalisation (**Figure 6**).

3.3.2.6 Serratus anterior free flap

Khan et al. published the first series utilising the serratus anterior free flap (SAFF) as an onlay to reinforce primary closure [55]. Authors cite the ease of harvest, low donor site morbidity, and the pliability of the flap as significant advantages over other free flaps used for similar purposes.

The shapes and sizes of all flaps depends upon the shape and size of the defect the surgeon is repairing.

3.4 Other considerations

3.4.1 Salivary bypass tube

The use of a salivary bypass tube to prevent PCF also remains controversial. While some maintain that salivary bypass tubes help funnel saliva into the oesophagus while bypassing the anastomosis, other denounce them as propagators of fistulation. Hone et al. found that in patients where a salivary bypass tube was used, the fistula rate was 8.3% compared to 24.6% in the control group [56]. However, in their multivariate analysis, this difference was not borne out to be significant. Perhaps the benefit of salivary bypass tubes in the circumferential reconstructive setting includes splinting of an otherwise highly collapsable neopharynx.

3.4.2 Tracheo-oesophageal puncture

Elective trachea-oesophageal puncture results in a fistula that allows for the use of a device for producing speech without reflux of digestive tract secretions into the trachea. The timing of tracheo-oesophageal puncture (TEP) placement is critical in the setting of salvage laryngectomy. Emerick et al. showed in salvage laryngectomy patients that fluency was 62 days earlier with the primary TEP group. However, the

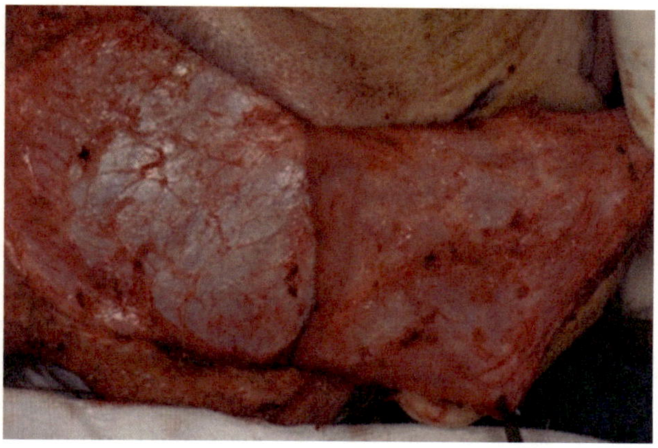

Figure 6.
Temporoparietal flap.

rate of PCF was also significantly higher in the primary TEP group (50%) versus in the secondary TEP group (0%) [57].

Our preference is to delay TEP in the setting of pharyngolaryngectomy until after discharge. We have found that the posterior wall of the trachea is prone to unpredictable and inadvertent dilatation which may result in a fistula that is too large and can make placement of a speaking device difficult.

4. Post-op considerations

4.1 Postoperative monitoring

Postoperative free flap monitoring protocols are highly variable among different institutions. A systematic review by Dort et al. [58] suggested the need for intensive monitoring in the first 24 hours as most evidence suggests that vascular complications will occur within the first 24 hours in most patients [59]. The method of monitoring should include clinical examination by experienced staff and adjunct measures, such as the use of ultrasound doppler and needle prick. As free tissue transfers are employed to salvage pharyngeal defects, the surrounding recipient vessels are frequently compromised, especially in the neck region. Our experiences indicate that the rate of free flap complications is much higher, and that it may be worsened by the post-operative catabolic state and any underlying comorbid diseases. Preoperative preparations are critical for these cases.

Postoperative nutritional support in the form of nasogastric (NG) tube feeding is common for patients undergoing major head and neck surgery. In the event of a laryngopharyngectomy, the NG tube may be placed via the tracheostome for later replacement with a trachea-oesophageal fistula (TOF) for voice rehabilitation. Feeding gastrostomy or jejunostomy tube insertion needs to be considered during the preoperative planning phase when prolonged nutritional support is expected [60].

4.2 General care of the complex head and neck reconstruction patient

4.2.1 Antimicrobials

Clean-contaminated head and neck oncologic cases have significantly higher perioperative wound infection rates compared to clean cases [61]. Antibiotics given one to two hours preoperatively are shown to reduce wound infection rate [62]. However, a longer duration of post-operative antibiotics (i.e. up to 5 days) has not shown increased benefit in either wound infection or pneumonia [63]. Upper aerodigestive tract decontamination also has not demonstrated significant benefit [64]. A sensible approach is to provide perioperative antibiotics for at least 48 hours postoperatively, and up to 5 days in the salvage setting.

4.2.2 Thyroid function

Thyroid function is reduced in most cases due to either thyroidectomy or radiation-induced thyroid injury. The predominant morphological changes consist of atrophy, chronic inflammation with lymphocytic infiltration, vascular fibrosis, and follicular hyperplasia [65]. Apart from itsthe direct effects on sympathetic activities, thyroid function has a crucial role in wound healing. It is therefore imperative that thyroid function is checked in salvage setting even if the patient has a residual thyroid gland.

4.2.3 Nutrition

Although head and neck cancer-specific enhanced recovery after surgery (ERAS) protocols are yet to be defined, the recommendations may be extrapolated from those of other surgical oncology populations. ERAS protocols include reduced fasting time, avoidance of dehydration, and preoperative carbohydrate loading [66]. The benefit of preoperative nutritional management is augmented by postoperative nutritional formulae, including immune-supportive "immunonutrition." Systematic reviews suggest a positive association between reduced length of hospital stay and postoperative administration of immunonutrition support [67]. Clinical studies explicitly targeting patients with pharyngeal reconstruction are warranted.

4.2.4 Cardiorespiratory rehab (and prehab)

Respiratory complications after major head and neck reconstruction may jeopardise postoperative recovery. Increased sputum load will delay the decannulation of tracheostomy and increase the overall length of stay [68]. Currently, there is no specific data available, but the benefit of respiratory physiotherapy is shown to have a clear benefit in general surgery postoperative setting [69]. Furthermore, improved recall has been demonstrated in a randomised study in head and neck patients who received preoperative education [70]. Introduction of breathing exercises as part of preoperative education would be beneficial.

4.3 Wound issues

4.3.1 Pharyngocutaenous fistula

Previous radiotherapy, previous chemotherapy, advanced primary tumours, concurrent neck dissection, and hypothyroidism are among the identified risk factors for developing a PCF [71]. With primary closure, the rate of PCF approximates 30–40% in most case series [42]. It incurs a number of effects including prolonged hospital stay, more intensive nursing and wound care requirements, delays to oral intake, delays in voice restoration, additional surgical procedures needed to address the fistula, gastrostomy-tube insertion, as well as catastrophic complications such as carotid and jugular bleeding [25].

A large case series showed that those who had received previous chemoradiotherapies had significantly higher incidences of wound complications (45 vs. 25%) and PCF rate (32 vs. 12%) when compared to those undergoing surgery without any previous therapy [72]. Consequently, the RTOG-91-11 study reported a major wound complication rate of 60% and a PCF rate of 30% in patients who underwent salvage laryngectomy [73].

The dual paddle technique was found to be protective against PCF formation [74]. It is important to note that three-quarters of the patients with PCF were managed successfully with conservative management, which suggests that repeated surgical intervention may be ill-advised, especially when there are concerns of poor wound healing from previous radiotherapy [30].

Dirven et al. [75] reported an association between fistula incidence and the interval between radiotherapy and surgery. There was a distinct difference in the incidence rates in patients who underwent salvage surgery within 12 months of radiotherapy (48%) and more than 12 months after radiotherapy (0%).

4.3.2 Wound sepsis and negative pressure dressing

The resection and donor site wounds must be cared for in patients with pharyngeal reconstruction. A systematic review showed no one dressing to be superior in primarily closed wounds [76]. The evidence for vacuum-assisted closure (VAC) device for complex open cervical wounds demonstrated a potential benefit [77]. Higher wound complication rates in salvage surgery would necessitate a more frequent use of VAC dressing after dehiscence and wound debridement.

4.3.3 Carotid blowout

Carotid blowout refers to the rupture of the carotid artery associated with neck surgery or radiation. It is uncommon but rapidly fatal. Radiotherapy results in a significantly higher rate of wound breakdown, PCF, and infection. Stripping of the carotid sheath, bacterial infection, and salivary contamination all contribute to desiccation and erosion of the carotid walls [78].

4.4 Donor site

Donor site morbidity is shown to be equivocal between free flap and pedicled flap reconstructions with no differences in the rate of infection, dehiscence, and haematoma [79]. The degree of functional impairment depends on the amount of tissue transferred as well as the patient's laterality.

4.5 Deglutition

Patients with the hypopharyngeal disease appear to have a significantly higher incidence of dysphagia [30]. This phenomenon is likely due to a loss of intrinsic propulsion and natural pharyngeal mucosa in the neopharynx [80]. Swallow studies are performed postoperatively between day 7 to day 10. Non-ionic water-soluble contrast (i.e. omnipaque 300) is used to reduce the risk of pneumonitis in case of aspiration [81]. Anastomotic integrity is assessed during fluoroscopy before initiation of oral intake.

4.6 Speech

There are two predominant types of alaryngeal speech for use after laryngectomy. Tracheo-oesophageal puncture (TEP) speech produces voice via passage of air from the lungs through a prosthetic valve positioned in the wall between the trachea and the pharynx or the upper oesophagus.. Oesophageal speech is achieved by passage of air from the mouth into the gastrointestinal track, which is oscillated through the oesophagus with simultaneous articulation of words. Voice produced by TEP is generally accepted as superior to oesophageal speech because TEP speech is lungpowered speech and, as such, may offer more durable and louder speech than oesophageal speech. Both primary and secondary punctures have shown success in achieving speech fluency [57, 82].

Speech quality was better with free flap than with PM flap reconstruction for oral cavity defects. However both free flap and PM flap reconstructions scored similarly on global quality of life, pain, swallowing, chewing, speech, activity, recreation, taste, saliva, anxiety, and on the composite score [79].

In gastric pull-up and jejunal flaps, while the puncture has been shown to be successful, the voice quality is often poor with a gurgling quality when compared to skin-lined flaps [29].

4.7 Role of specialised nursing postoperatively to coordinate recovery

The perioperative complexity of pharyngeal reconstruction extends well beyond the confines of the operating room. Specialised nursing staff are required for continuity of care, troubleshooting of early signs of deterioration, and the co-ordination of airway, chest, feeding, and rehabilitation priorities. Historically, roles of nursing staff centred on head and neck surgical patients [83] originated when specialist nursing team began managing increasing numbers of these patients on nonsurgical wards. These patient wards were described as "Critical Care Outreach teams" [84]. This ward specialises and focuses on the management of complex head and neck patients. The support provided by specialist nurses has contributed to decreases in complication rates, readmissions to the ICU, and the overall length of stay [85].

5. Conclusion

The pharyngeal defect poses challenges to reconstructive surgeons, especially when the patient has a hostile neck from previous surgery or radiotherapy. The reconstruction plan needs to be patient- and defect- oriented. The surgeon should carefully consider the available options to achieve most, if not all, of the reconstructive goals. Complex head and neck surgical patients also require a team of specialised professionals to assist in their journey of healing and recovery. Such a multidisciplinary team is a crucial part of reintegration of cancer survivors back to society.

Conflict of interest

Authors declare that there are no conflicts of interest.

Appendices and nomenclature

ALT	anterolateral thigh
ERAS	enhanced recovery after surgery
HPV	human papillomavirus
PCF	pharyngocutaneous fistula
PM	pectoralis major

RFFF	radial forearm free flap
SAFF	serratus anterior free flap
SCAIF	supraclavicular artery island flap
SCC	squamous cell carcinoma
TAA	thoracoacrominal artery perforator
TCA	transcervical artery
TEP	tracheoesophageal puncture
TOF	trachea-oesophageal fistula
TORS	transoral robotic surgery
TPFF	temporoparietal fascial free flap
VAC	vacuum-assisted closure

Author details

Takako Yabe[1] and Bruce Ashford[1,2]*

1 Illawarra Shoalhaven Local Health District, NSW, Australia

2 University of Wollongong, Australia

*Address all correspondence to: bruceash@uow.edu.au

References

[1] Lefebvre JL, Andry G, Chevalier D, Luboinski B, Collette L, Traissac L, et al. Laryngeal preservation with induction chemotherapy for hypopharyngeal squamous cell carcinoma: 10-year results of EORTC trial 24891. Annals of Oncology. 2012;**23**(10):2708-2714

[2] Caliceti U, Sgarzani R, Cipriani R, Cantore S, Contedini F, Pinto V, et al. Single stage reconstruction of complex head and neck defects involving the skin with a single ALT flap: A ten year review. Journal of Plastic, Reconstructive and Aesthetic Surgery. 2019;**22**:55-64

[3] Department of Veterans Affairs Laryngeal Cancer Study G, Wolf GT, Fisher SG, Hong WK, Hillman R, Spaulding M, et al. Induction chemotherapy plus radiation compared with surgery plus radiation in patients with advanced laryngeal cancer. The New England Journal of Medicine. 1991;**324**(24):1685-1690

[4] Forastiere AA, Zhang Q, Weber RS, Maor MH, Goepfert H, Pajak TF, et al. Long-term results of RTOG 91-11: A comparison of three nonsurgical treatment strategies to preserve the larynx in patients with locally advanced larynx cancer. Journal of Clinical Oncology. 2013;**31**(7):845-852

[5] Agrawal N, Goldenberg D. Primary and salvage total laryngectomy. Otolaryngologic Clinics of North America. 2008;**41**(4):771-780 vii

[6] Mäkitie AA, Irish J, Gullane PJ. Pharyngocutaneous fistula. Current Opinion in Otolaryngology & Head and Neck Surgery. 2003;**11**(2):78-84

[7] Disa JJ, Cordeiro PG. Reconstruction of the hypopharynx and cervical esophagus. Clinics in Plastic Surgery. 2001;**28**(2):349-360

[8] Sumer BD, Gastman BR, Nussenbaum B, Gao F, Haughey BH. Microvascular flap reconstruction of major pharyngeal resections with the intent of laryngeal preservation. Archives of Otolaryngology--Head & Neck Surgery. 2009;**135**(8):801-806

[9] Penel N, Fournier C, Lefebvre D, Roussel-Delvallez M, Sarini J, Kara A, et al. Previous chemotherapy as a predictor of wound infections in nonmajor head and neck surgery: Results of a prospective study. Head & Neck. 2004;**26**(6):513-517

[10] Fung K, Teknos TN, Vandenberg CD, Lyden TH, Bradford CR, Hogikyan ND, et al. Prevention of wound complications following salvage laryngectomy using free vascularized tissue. Head & Neck. 2007;**29**(5):425-430

[11] McGurk M, Goodger N. Head and neck cancer and its treatment: Historical review. British Journal of Oral and Maxillofacial Surgery. 2000;**38**(3):209-220

[12] Tamai S. History of microsurgery. Plastics and Reconstructive Surgery. 2009;**124**(6S):e282-e294

[13] Jiang N, Zhang LJ, Li LY, Zhao Y, Eisele DW. Risk factors for late dysphagia after (chemo)radiotherapy for head and neck cancer: A systematic methodological review. Head & Neck. 2016;**38**(5):792-800

[14] Mahalingam S, Srinivasan R, Spielmann P. Quality-of-life and functional outcomes following pharyngolaryngectomy: A systematic review of literature. Clinical Otolaryngology. 2016;**41**(1):25-43

[15] Takes RP, Strojan P, Silver CE, Bradley PJ, Haigentz M Jr, Wolf GT, et al. Current trends in initial management of

hypopharyngeal cancer: The declining use of open surgery. Head & Neck. 2012;**34**(2):270-281

[16] Disa JJ, Pusic AL, Mehrara BJ. Reconstruction of the hypopharynx with the free jejunum transfer. Journal of Surgical Oncology. 2006;**94**(6):466-470

[17] Ferahkose Z, Bedirli A, Kerem M, Azili C, Sozuer EM, Akin M. Comparison of free jejunal graft with gastric pull-up reconstruction after resection of hypopharyngeal and cervical esophageal carcinoma. Diseases of the Esophagus. 2008;**21**(4):340-345

[18] Nouraei SA, Mace AD, Middleton SE, Hudovsky A, Vaz F, Moss C, et al. A stratified analysis of the perioperative outcome of 17623 patients undergoing major head and neck cancer surgery in England over 10 years: Towards an informatics-based outcomes surveillance framework. Clinical Otolaryngology. 2017;**42**(1):11-28

[19] Patel SY, Meram AT, Kim DD. Soft tissue reconstruction for head and neck ablative defects. Oral and Maxillofacial Surgery Clinics of North America. 2019;**31**(1):39-68

[20] Couch ME. Laryngopharyngectomy with reconstruction. Otolaryngologic Clinics of North America. 2002;**35**(5):1097-1114

[21] Chan YW, Ng RW, Liu LH, Chung HP, Wei WI. Reconstruction of circumferential pharyngeal defects after tumour resection: Reference or preference. Journal of Plastic, Reconstructive and Aesthetic Surgery. 2011;**64**(8):1022-1028

[22] Chim H, Salgado CJ, Seselgyte R, Wei F-C, Mardini S, editors. Principles of Head and Neck Reconstruction: An Algorithm to Guide Flap Selection. Seminars in Plastic Surgery. Thieme Medical Publishers; 2010

[23] Kelly KE, Anthony JP, Singer M. Pharyngoesophageal reconstruction using the radial forearm fasciocutaneous free flap: Preliminary results. Otolaryngology–Head and Neck Surgery. 1994;**111**(1):16-24

[24] Novakovic D, Patel RS, Goldstein DP, Gullane PJ. Salvage of failed free flaps used in head and neck reconstruction. Head & Neck Oncology. 2009;**1**(1):33

[25] Yeh DH, Sahovaler A, Fung K. Reconstruction after salvage laryngectomy. Oral Oncology. 2017;**75**:22-27

[26] Hui Y, Wei WI, Yuen PW, Lam LK, Ho WK. Primary closure of pharyngeal remnant after total laryngectomy and partial pharyngectomy: How much residual mucosa is sufficient? The Laryngoscope. 1996;**106**(4):490-494

[27] Sassler AM, Esclamado RM, Wolf GT. Surgery after organ preservation therapy. Analysis of wound complications. Archives of Otolaryngology--Head & Neck Surgery. 1995;**121**(2):162-165

[28] Su CY, Chiang YC. The fabricated radial forearm flap in pharyngolaryngeal surgery: Saliva leakage and its prevention. British Journal of Plastic Surgery. 1995;**48**(4):212-217

[29] Cho BC, Kim M, Lee JH, Byun JS, Park JS, Baik BS. Pharyngoesophageal reconstruction with a tubed free radial forearm flap. Journal of Reconstructive Microsurgery. 1998;**14**(8):535-540

[30] Balasubramanian D, Subramaniam N, Rathod P, Murthy S, Sharma M, Mathew J, et al. Outcomes following pharyngeal reconstruction in total laryngectomy - institutional experience and review of literature. Indian Journal of Plastic Surgery. 2018;**51**(2):190-195

[31] Ariyan S. The pectoralis major myocutaneous flap. A versatile flap for reconstruction in the head and neck. Plastic and Reconstructive Surgery. 1979;**63**(1):73-81

[32] Patel UA, Moore BA, Wax M, Rosenthal E, Sweeny L, Militsakh ON, et al. Impact of pharyngeal closure technique on fistula after salvage laryngectomy. JAMA Otolaryngology-Head & Neck Surgery. 2013;**139**(11):1156-1162

[33] Burke MS, Kaplan SE, Kaplowitz LJ, Lotempio MM, Hicks WL Jr, Rigual NR, et al. Pectoralis major myocutaneous flap for reconstruction of circumferential pharyngeal defects. Annals of Plastic Surgery. 2013;**71**(6):649-651

[34] Deschler DG, Doherty ET, Reed CG, Singer MI. Quantitative and qualitative analysis of tracheoesophageal voice after pectoralis major flap reconstruction of the neopharynx. Otolaryngology–Head and Neck Surgery. 1998;**118**(6):771-776

[35] Emerick KS, Herr MA, Deschler DG. Supraclavicular flap reconstruction following total laryngectomy. The Laryngoscope. 2014;**124**(8):1777-1782

[36] Trautman J, Gore S, Potter M, Clark J, Hyam D, Tan NC, et al. Supraclavicular flap repair in the free flap era. ANZ Journal of Surgery. 2018;**88**(6):540-546

[37] Lamberty BGH. The supra-clavicular axial patterned flap. British Journal of Plastic Surgery. 1979;**32**(3):207-212

[38] Iyer NG, Clark JR, Ashford BG. Internal mammary artery perforator flap for head and neck reconstruction. ANZ Journal of Surgery. 2009;**79**(11):799-803

[39] Song D, Pafitanis G, Pont LEP, Yang P, Koshima I, Zhang Y, et al. Chimeric thoracoacromial artery perforator flap for one-staged reconstruction of complex pharyngoesophageal defects: A single unit experience. Head & Neck. 2018;**40**(2):302-311

[40] Sayles M, Grant DG. Preventing pharyngo-cutaneous fistula in total laryngectomy: A systematic review and meta-analysis. The Laryngoscope. 2014;**124**(5):1150-1163

[41] Higgins KM, Ashford B, Erovic BM, Yoo J, Enepekides DJ. Temporoparietal fascia free flap for pharyngeal coverage after salvage total laryngectomy. The Laryngoscope. 2012;**122**(3):523-527

[42] Paleri V, Drinnan M, Van Den Brekel MW, Hinni ML, Bradley PJ, Wolf GT, et al. Vascularized tissue to reduce fistula following salvage total laryngectomy: A systematic review. The Laryngoscope. 2014;**124**(8):1848-1853

[43] Azizzadeh B, Yafai S, Rawnsley JD, Abemayor E, Sercarz JA, Calcaterra TC, et al. Radial forearm free flap pharyngoesophageal reconstruction. The Laryngoscope. 2001;**111**(5):807-810

[44] Nojima K, Brown SA, Acikel C, Arbique G, Ozturk S, Chao J, et al. Defining vascular supply and territory of thinned perforator flaps: Part I. anterolateral thigh perforator flap. Plastic and Reconstructive Surgery. 2005;**116**(1):182-193

[45] Zelken JA, Kang CJ, Huang SF, Liao CT, Tsao CK. Refinements in flap design and inset for pharyngoesophageal reconstruction with free thigh flaps. Microsurgery. 2017;**37**(2):112-118

[46] Wong CH, Wei FC. Microsurgical free flap in head and neck reconstruction. Head & Neck. 2010;**32**(9):1236-1245

[47] Benazzo M, Occhini A, Fossati G, Caracciolo G. Reconstruction of intrathoracic oesophagus using tubular lateral thigh free flap. The Journal of Laryngology and Otology. 2000;**114**(7):551-553

[48] Baudet J. Reconstruction of the pharyngeal wall by free transfer of the greater omentum and stomach. International Journal of Microsurgery. 1979;**1**:53-59

[49] Craig SJ, Zhang A, Gardner TD, Clark JR, Ashford BG. Laparoscopic harvest of the gastro-omental free flap for reconstruction after total pharyngolaryngectomy: Operative technique. Head & Neck. 2017

[50] Patel RS, Gilbert RW. Utility of the gastro-omental free flap in head and neck reconstruction. Current Opinion in Otolaryngology & Head and Neck Surgery. 2009;**17**(4):258-262

[51] Moran WJ, Panje WR. The free greater omental flap for treatment of mandibular osteoradionecrosis. Archives of Otolaryngology--Head & Neck Surgery. 1987;**113**(4):425-427

[52] Perez-Smith D, Wagels M, Theile DR. Jejunal free flap reconstruction of the pharyngolaryngectomy defect: 368 consecutive cases. Journal of Plastic, Reconstructive and Aesthetic Surgery. 2013;**66**(1):9-15

[53] Bearelly S, Heaton CM, Seth R, Daniel KP. Laryngopharyngeal repair in salvage Laryngectomy. Current Otorhinolaryngology Reports. 2016;**4**(3):211-218

[54] van Brederode TD, Halmos GB, Stenekes MW. Functional outcome after one-stage flap reconstruction of the hypopharynx following tumor ablation. European Archives of Oto-Rhino-Laryngology. 2017;**274**(2):969-976

[55] Khan MN, Rodriguez LG, Pool CD, Laitman B, Hernandez C, Erovic BM, et al. The versatility of the serratus anterior free flap in head and neck reconstruction. The Laryngoscope. 2017;**127**(3):568-573

[56] Hone RWA, Rahman E, Wong G, Annan Y, Alexander V, Al-Lami A, et al. Do salivary bypass tubes lower the incidence of pharyngocutaneous fistula following total laryngectomy? A retrospective analysis of predictive factors using multivariate analysis. European Archives of Oto-Rhino-Laryngology. 2017;**274**(4):1983-1991

[57] Emerick KS, Tomycz L, Bradford CR, Lyden TH, Chepeha DB, Wolf GT, et al. Primary versus secondary tracheoesophageal puncture in salvage total laryngectomy following chemoradiation. Otolaryngology–Head and Neck Surgery. 2009;**140**(3):386-390

[58] Dort JC, Farwell DG, Findlay M, Huber GF, Kerr P, Shea-Budgell MA, et al. Optimal perioperative Care in Major Head and Neck Cancer Surgery with Free Flap Reconstruction: A consensus review and recommendations from the enhanced recovery after surgery society. JAMA Otolaryngology-Head & Neck Surgery. 2017;**143**(3):292-303

[59] Pattani KM, Byrne P, Boahene K, Richmon J. What makes a good flap go bad? A critical analysis of the literature of intraoperative factors related to free flap failure. The Laryngoscope. 2010;**120**(4):717-723

[60] Talwar B, Findlay M. When is the optimal time for placing a gastrostomy in patients undergoing treatment for head and neck cancer? Current Opinion in Supportive and Palliative Care. 2012;**6**(1):41-53

[61] Skitarelić N, Morović M, Manestar D. Antibiotic prophylaxis in clean-contaminated head and neck

oncological surgery. Journal of Cranio-Maxillofacial surgery. 2007;**35**(1):15-20

[62] Rodrigo JP, Alvarez JC, Gómez JR, Suárez C, Fernández JA, Martínez JA. Comparison of three prophylactic antibiotic regimens in clean-contaminated head and neck surgery. Head & neck. 1997;**19**(3):188-193

[63] Liu SA, Tung KC, Shiao JY, Chiu YT. Preliminary report of associated factors in wound infection after major head and neck neoplasm operations--does the duration of prophylactic antibiotic matter? The Journal of Laryngology & Otology. 2008;**122**(4):403-408

[64] Simons JP, Johnson JT, Yu VL, Vickers RM, Gooding WE, Myers EN, et al. The role of topical antibiotic prophylaxis in patients undergoing contaminated head and neck surgery with flap reconstruction. The Laryngoscope. 2001;**111**(2):329-335

[65] Galbo AML, Kuik DJ, Lips P, von Blomberg BME, Bloemena E, Leemans CR, et al. A prospective longitudinal study on endocrine dysfunction following treatment of laryngeal or hypopharyngeal carcinoma. Oral Oncology. 2013;**49**(9):950-955

[66] Mortensen K, Nilsson M, Slim K, Schäfer M, Mariette C, Braga M, et al. Consensus guidelines for enhanced recovery after gastrectomy: Enhanced recovery after surgery (ERAS®) society recommendations. British Journal of Surgery. 2014;**101**(10):1209-1229

[67] Drover JW, Dhaliwal R, Weitzel L, Wischmeyer PE, Ochoa JB, Heyland DK. Perioperative use of arginine-supplemented diets: A systematic review of the evidence. Journal of the American College of Surgeons. 2011;**212**(3):385-399, 399.e381

[68] Brookes JT, Seikaly H, Diamond C, Mechor B, Harris JR. Prospective randomized trial comparing the effect of early suturing of tracheostomy sites on postoperative patient swallowing and rehabilitation. Journal of Otolaryngology. 2006;**35**(2):77-82

[69] Thomas JA, McIntosh JM. Are incentive spirometry, intermittent positive pressure breathing, and deep breathing exercises effective in the prevention of postoperative pulmonary complications after upper abdominal surgery? A systematic overview and meta-analysis. Physical Therapy. 1994;**74**(1):3-10 discussion 10-16

[70] Chan Y, Irish JC, Wood SJ, Rotstein LE, Brown DH, Gullane PJ, et al. Patient education and informed consent in head and neck surgery. Archives of Otolaryngology--Head & Neck Surgery. 2002;**128**(11):1269-1274

[71] Dedivitis RA, Aires FT, Cernea CR, Brandão LG. Pharyngocutaneous fistula after total laryngectomy: Systematic review of risk factors. Head & Neck. 2015;**37**(11):1691-1697

[72] Ganly I, Patel S, Matsuo J, Singh B, Kraus D, Boyle J, et al. Postoperative complications of salvage total laryngectomy. Cancer. 2005;**103**(10):2073-2081

[73] Forastiere AA, Goepfert H, Maor M, Pajak TF, Weber R, Morrison W, et al. Concurrent chemotherapy and radiotherapy for organ preservation in advanced laryngeal cancer. The New England Journal of Medicine. 2003;**349**(22):2091-2098

[74] Sparks DS, Myers H, Grinsell D. Single-stage reconstruction of combined hypopharyngeal and anterior neck skin defects with the dual-paddle anterolateral thigh flap. European Journal of Plastic Surgery. 2018;**41**(3):299-306

[75] Dirven R, Swinson BD, Gao K, Clark JR. The assessment

of pharyngocutaneous fistula rate in patients treated primarily with definitive radiotherapy followed by salvage surgery of the larynx and hypopharynx. The Laryngoscope. 2009;**119**(9):1691-1695

[76] Dumville JC, Gray TA, Walter CJ, Sharp CA, Page T, Macefield R, et al. Dressings for the prevention of surgical site infection. Cochrane Database of Systematic Reviews. 2016;**12**

[77] Satteson ES, Crantford JC, Wood J, David LR. Outcomes of vacuum-assisted therapy in the treatment of head and neck wounds. The Journal of Craniofacial Surgery. 2015;**26**(7):e599-e602

[78] Suárez C, Fernández-Alvarez V, Hamoir M, Mendenhall WM, Strojan P, Quer M, et al. Carotid blowout syndrome: Modern trends in management. Cancer Management and Research. 2018;**10**:5617

[79] Gabrysz-Forget F, Tabet P, Rahal A, Bissada E, Christopoulos A, Ayad T. Free versus pedicled flaps for reconstruction of head and neck cancer defects: A systematic review. Journal of Otolaryngology - Head & Neck Surgery. 2019;**48**(1):13

[80] Walther EK, Herberhold C. Computerized manometry and deglutition after pharyngolaryngeal tumor resections. Laryngo- Rhino-Otologie. 1993;**72**(2):67-72

[81] Zhong J, Nejadhamzeeigilani H, Thomson E, Tolan D, Roe G, Kaye T, editors. Fluoroscopy at its Finest: Post-Operative Assessment after Laryngo-Pharyngeal and Upper Gastrointestinal Tract surgery2017. European Congress of Radiology; 2017

[82] Gitomer SA, Hutcheson KA, Christianson BL, Samuelson MB, Barringer DA, Roberts DB, et al. Influence of timing, radiation, and reconstruction on complications and speech outcomes with tracheoesophageal puncture. Head & Neck. 2016;**38**(12):1765-1771

[83] Russell C, Harkin H. The benefits of tracheostomy specialist nurses. Nursing Times. 2001;**97**(46):40

[84] Lewis T, Oliver G. Improving tracheostomy care for ward patients. Nursing Standard. 2005;**19**(19):33

[85] Sodhi K, Shrivastava A, Singla MK. Implications of dedicated tracheostomy care nurse program on outcomes. Journal of Anesthesia. 2014;**28**(3):374-380

Chapter 4

Commonly Utilized Non Vascularised Bone Grafts in Maxillofacial Reconstruction

Manish Anand and Shreya Panwar

Abstract

Surgical defects created secondary to oncological resection are often debilitating for patients, both functionally and esthetically. Meticulous surgical planning and intricate knowledge of the vital anatomical structures are essential for understanding the biology of reconstruction in the craniofacial skeleton. Unlike reconstructive procedures in other areas where the functional components may be given priority, reconstruction of the face requires a delicate balance between the esthetic and functional units. Despite new developments, autogenous grafts have frequently remained a reliable alternative that withstood the test of time. Non-vascularized bone grafts are often a subset of autogenous grafts, where the graft solely depends on the recipient's vascularity and is indicated in defect sizes of less than 6 cm.

Keywords: non vascularized bone graft, maxillofacial surgery, critical defect, cortico-cancellous graft

1. Introduction

Resection and reconstruction are two vital components of surgical oncology. While the former depends primarily on the surgeon's discretion, the latter includes a vital role for the patient. The surgical team must consider the patient's desired outcome (especially in terms of facial esthetics) and remain cautious of critical aspects such as early bone resorption, infection and donor site morbidity.

The first bone graft dates back to 1881 when Sir William MacEwan performed a successful xenograft transfer into a craniofacial defect [1]. Currently, common non-vascularized bone graft (NVBG) options include anterior or posterior iliac crest, cranial vault and costochondral grafts [2]. Multiple studies had demonstrated a relatively high success rate between 85–90% when NVBG were used regardless of the type of injury [3–5].

Bone defects in the craniomaxillofacial complex require three-dimensional structural considerations to ensure proper dental occlusion and temporomandibular joint function. This makes any reconstructive surgery in the craniomaxillofacial skeleton complex and challenging [5, 6]. In most such reconstructions, fresh autogenous bone is the gold standard bone grafting material [7]. There are three typical ways in which fresh autogenous graft can be transferred:

IntechOpen

- Non-vascularized grafts,
- Pedicled grafts, and
- Microvascular free flaps.

2. Concept of a 'critical-sized bone defect'

In simple terms, a critical-sized bone defect is the minimum size defect beyond which bone fails to heal spontaneously despite surgical fixation, requiring further surgical intervention [8]. It is imperative to diagnose critical-sized bone defect as this will help surgeons decide the need for surgical intervention [9]. Although there is no clear-cut consensus in the literature regarding minimum defect size measurement, a few studies have estimated this value to be in the range of 4 mm–5 mm [8, 9]. Defect size less than this measurement can be managed by plate and screw fixation, but anything above this value must be considered for grafting and subsequent fixation [8–10].

3. Factors to be considered before bone grafting

- Age of the patient - Older individuals have decreased healing capacities as compared to the younger groups. Moreover, systemic complications such as diabetes, hypertension, and cardiovascular diseases are more common in geriatric patients and must be ruled out [11]. Surgical reinforcements like the bone morphogenic protein (BMP-2) or plasma rich platelet therapy should be considered to promote faster healing [11–13].

- Nature of the disease – NVBG is primarily indicated in benign lesions where the risks of recurrence are low as it aids in better graft uptake. Furthermore, malignant lesions are frequently treated with radiotherapy, which compromises the capacity for angiogenesis into grafted tissues [5, 14].

- Size of the defect – As previously mentioned, 5 cm is the maximum defect size that can be reconstructed with NVBG. Beyond 5 cm, a graft needs its own blood supply in the form of a vascularized graft as NVBG depends solely on recipient site vasculature [15, 16].

- Need for adjuvant Radiotherapy_– Radiation causes compromises blood supply and cellular function in recipient tissue beds. According to the current guidelines of management of head and neck pathologies, NVBG should not be the first choice in patients who require radiation therapy. If radiation is planned, it should be administered at least six months before and after grafting to ensure that the graft develops an adequate blood supply [17].

- Timing of reconstruction – Surgical intervention may occur as a single- or two-staged operation. The single-staged modality refers to immediate reconstruction after ablation. This allows for shorter duration of treatment and maintenance of pre-operative soft tissue contours. On the other hand, the two-staged modality refers to initial ablation followed by reconstruction at a later date. This provides ample time for planning the reconstruction.

The authors favor immediate grafting as it averts the need for a second surgery and minimizes the total treatment duration.

- Type of bone required – Cortical bone resists resorption and maintains its structural integrity post-operatively. Conversely, cancellous bone is more porous and demonstrates a faster rate of resorption. However, there is also rapid neovascularization in cancellous bone when compared to cortical bone. Calvarial grafts have more cortical component, while the iliac crest has a more cancellous component [18, 19].

3.1 Graft donor sites

Following options are available to the surgical team in the reconstruction of maxillofacial defects

- Bone graft from anterior or posterior ileum
- Bone graft from calvarium
- Bone graft from tibia
- Bone graft from rib

4. Iliac crest bone graft

Autogenous bone harvested from the ileum serves as an excellent source of cortico-cancellous graft with a maximum harvest volume of 50 cc for the anterior iliac crest and 100 cc for the posterior iliac crest [2, 5]. In general, harvests from the anterior iliac region are considered easier and safer because they do not require intra-operative repositioning [7, 20].

The important anatomical landmarks that should be considered during surgery are the anterior superior iliac spine (ASIS) and iliac tubercle, which is 6 cm posterior to the ASIS. The iliac crest receives its blood supply from the deep circumflex iliac artery, a branch of the internal iliac artery and the most common bleeding source during surgery [7, 20, 21]. Sensory nerves that must be protected are iliohypogastric nerve and lateral femoral cutaneous nerve. The lateral femoral cutaneous nerve (LFCN) is at increased risk of damage during surgery and must be identified and protected from iatrogenic injuries. According to Mischowski et al. the LFCN courses between 5 to 14.6 mm superiolaterally from the ASIS [22, 23].

4.1 Anterior iliac bone harvest

A curvilinear incision is placed 2 cm superior to the ASIS along the iliac crest to prevent injury to the LFCN, and the dissection is taken down through subcutaneous tissue to the muscular levels. The external oblique muscle and tensor fascia lata are identified and lateralized to expose periosteum. The periosteum is then incised, and the iliacus muscle is identified and retracted medially [2, 7, 24]. Osteotomy is performed along the length of the iliac tubercle joined by two vertical cuts at the ends of the osteotomy along the medial iliac curvature. The cortical bone may be harvested with an osteotome and the cancellous bone using a bone gouge [2, 24]. There are various other approaches described in the literature for harvesting the anterior iliac crest. In the trapdoor approach, the medial or lateral bony cortex is pedicled with an attached muscle to gain visualization to the cancellous bone. The Tschopp technique involves obliquely osteotomizing the iliac crest. A third approach, the Tessier approach, involves medial and lateral oblique osteotomies to gain access to the underlying cancellous bone [25–27].

The trapdoor technique allows direct access to the cancellous bone while preserving the attachments to the muscle and abdominal fascia [26]. On the contrary, Tschopp and Tessier techniques preserve the natural contour of the iliac crest, improving post-operative cosmesis [24, 26, 27].

A maximum of 3 x 5 cm of cortical bone and 50 cc of cancellous bone [2, 23, 24] can be harvested from anterior ileum. This is typically sufficient to reconstruct mandibular segmental defect up to 5 cm [2, 6, 7].

4.2 Posterior iliac crest bone graft

The posterior ileum can provide up to 100 cc of corticocancellous, uncompressed bone [2, 6]. The posterior iliac crest also demonstrates extremely low rates of post-op morbidity including gait and neurosensory disturbances [2, 6, 27–29]. However, additional anesthetic risks are present associated with the prone position [2, 6, 28].

Relevant anatomy – The sacroiliac joint is the primary anatomical landmark. Just below the joint, the gluteus maximus muscle attaches to the triangular tubercle which measures approximately 3 x 4 cm. The superior and medial cluneal nerves arise from the dorsal rami of L1, L2 and L3 and lies approximately 6.5 cm from the posterior superior iliac spine (PSIS) [2, 6, 29]. Surgical approach to the posterior iliac graft begins in the prone position with 210-degree reverse hip flexion. The incision is designed 1 cm from the PSIS and carried 5–6 cm along the crest superolaterally to avoid injury to the cluneal nerves [2, 29]. Dissection is then carried out incising skin then subcutaneous tissues to the level of fascial attachments of the internal oblique and gluteus maximus muscles. The dissection is also performed between superior and middle cluneal nerves to expose the posterior iliac periosteam [6, 29]. Sharp incision of periosteum is then conducted using electrocautery taking care not to damage the sacroiliac ligaments. Depending on the graft volume requirement, an osteotomy may be made approximately 4 to 5 cm inferior to the iliac crest.

A 2012 study by Abramowicz et al. demonstrated that bone graft from the posterior iliac crest benefits from decreased blood loss and fewer post-op morbidities when compared to the anterior graft. On the contrary, intraoperative and anesthesia times were significantly lower in the anterior graft [30].

4.3 Complications

The most commonly documented complications in anterior iliac graft harvest are hematoma, seroma, gait disturbance, pelvic instability, persistent pain, abdominal pain, and infection [31, 32]. In their ten years of analysis, Antonio et al. reported predominantly minor complications that would frequently self-correct within five weeks [33]. Another study by Manar et al. of 372 patients reported only two major complications consisting of fracture and seroma [34]. Various authors have recommended the use of a reciprocating saw and to maintain a clear margin of at least 3 cm posterior to ASIS to prevent fracture of the iliac spine [2, 4, 26, 29].

Posterior iliac graft harvesting tends to have fewer complications which can include bleeding, ureteral injury, abdominal hernia, paresthesia, seroma and infection [32, 35]. Studies by Elke Ahlmann et al., Nkenke et al., and Mazock et al. concluded that harvesting of the posterior iliac graft is associated with a significantly lower number of complications [28, 36, 37].

Overall, bone harvest from the iliac region is general safe and provides an adequate amount of good quality cortico-cancellous bone.

5. Calvarial bone graft

Historically, calvarial bone is one of the most commonly harvested grafts in the reconstruction of craniofacial defects [2]. The calvarium shares a common embryological origin as the other bones of the maxillofacial region and develop through intramembranous ossification [2, 18]. As a result, they demonstrate slower resorption rates than many other NVBGs. The calvarial grafts are also advantageous in that they are frequently obtained from the same surgical field and that they are anatomically distant from critical structures like vessels and nerves. This allows the graft to be harvested with decreased morbidity and technicality [2, 38].

However, potential complications do exist including dural tears, post-operative structural deformity, alopecia, and an inadequate amount of cancellous bone [39]. The calvarial bone graft is particularly indicated where structural integrity is needed in reconstructions of the maxilla, nasal dorsum, zygomatic pillars, orbital floors and the frontal bone [2, 38, 40].

Relevant anatomy and surgical technique: Anatomically, the calvarium comprises of singular frontal and occipital bones as well as paired parietal and temporal bones. Calvarial bone grafts are best harvested from the parietal region that measures approximately 8x10 cm. The skull is made up of the outer cortex (cortical bone), the medullary space (cancellous bone), and inner cortex (cortical bone) all of which may be harvested for use [18]. Surgeons must remain diligent when approaching the inner cortex to avoid tears to the underlying dura covering the brain [2, 18]. Inadvertent dural injuries can lead to hematoma and/or CSF leakage. In a case series of 23 patients, Harsha et al. reported three cases of perforation of the inner cortex, one of which incurred dural tear that required primary closure [41]. Another anatomical limit that must be taken into account is the temporoparietal suture, as any osteotomy below this line risks intracranial exposure because of the thinness of the bone.

The calvarial bone graft may be taken at three different levels [38, 42]

i. Partial-thickness outer cortex: only a strip of the outer cortex is harvested. It is suitable for children between 4 to 6 years of age, especially in the reconstruction of craniofacial anomalies.

ii. Full-thickness outer cortex: whole outer cortex is harvested. This is more suitable for adult patients.

iii. Inner cortex: in some cases, where craniotomy has previously been performed, the inner cortex can be harvested leaving the outer cortex behind.

In cases where a broad area of reconstruction is required, the bicortical technique is preferred, where the two cortices are split, thereby doubling the graft's available surface area [42].

Surgical technique – The coronal incision is the most preferred technique as it allows a wide area of visualization to the underlying parietal bone. The incision starts from one helical crus to the other, approximately 2 to 3 cm posterior to hairline [2, 7, 42, 43]. Once the scalp flap is raised, an avascular plane is created between the pericranium and the galea, and the external surface of the skull is then exposed through subgaleal dissection. All osteotomies must be made at least 2 cm away from the temporoparietal and sagittal sutures. Venturing beyond these landmarks leads to increased risks of perforating the dural layer [38, 43, 44]. Based on the technique mentioned above, the surgeon may make the harvest using a Gigli saw and osteotome. Once a strip of bone is harvested, the defect may be filled with an alloplastic substitute that helps maintain the natural contour of the skull. The closure is then performed in layers, and a pressure pack is applied for 48–72 hours [2, 38, 43, 44].

5.1 Complications

Complications related to calvarial harvests are few and depend on the technique performed. The bi-cortical harvesting technique significantly increases the risk of complications because it interferes with the inner cortex, which lies close to the dural layer [2, 42]. In a study by Frodel et al. 3 cases of dural tear were reported in 121 patients who underwent bicortical grafts, of which 2 were less than 1 cm and required minimum intervention. In one case, however, there was an intracerebral injury, requiring neurosurgical intervention [38]. In another study of 511 cases by Sandrine Touzet et al., 13 cases of immediate complications were noted, including 2 cases of hematoma of the scalp and 11 cases of dural exposure. Late complications occurred in 12 patients with alopecia, 2 with residual pain, 8 with dysesthesia, and 420 with skull depression [45].

Most dural complications may be avoided via the use of pre-operative computed tomography to measure the thickness of the parietal bones [2, 7, 38–44]. Post-op skull depressions may also be addressed via secondary alloplastic grafting [46]. With increasing sophistication of practice, the number of complications associated with calvarial bone grafts has dropped significantly in the past few years.

6. Tibial bone graft

Bone harvested from the proximal tibia is an excellent source of cancellous bone, which is helpful in addressing "spacial defects" like pneumatized maxillary sinuses and 3 to 4 osseous wall defects [47]. This procedure is generally indicated in adults where skeletal maturity has been achieved [2, 47, 48]. The amount of cancellous bone obtained from the tibia is approximately 20 cc, somewhat less than the bone obtainable at the anterior iliac crest. Bone grafts from the tibia can be harvested either from the medial or the lateral side, but the lateral approach is preferred because of a decreased rate of complications [2, 47].

Relevant anatomy – The most important anatomical landmark for the lateral approach of harvesting tibial bone graft is Gerdy's tubercle [2, 7, 47, 49]. It is the insertion site of the iliotibialis tract on the proximal and the lateral aspects of the tibia. Gerdy's tubercle is a bony prominence and is a key marker to be noted before placing an incision [49]. Other anatomical landmarks include the patella, patellar ligament, tibial tuberosity, and the fibular head, which includes Gerdy's tubercle. The lateral cutaneous branch of the sural nerve frequently crosses over Gerdy's tubercle and the surgeon must remain diligent while dissecting along the course of this nerve. Small terminal branches of the inferior genicular and the recurrent anterior tibial arteries may also cross Gerdy's tubercle, which can be readily cauterized during surgery [47]. Avoidance of major neurovascular structures is done with relative ease, rending the proximal tibia a safe alternative harvest site [7, 47].

Surgical technique – Identification of Gerdy's tubercle is the key step of this technique. Once identified and confirmed with palpation, a 3–4 cm incision is made directly over the tubercle. The incision is then continued to the periosteum, which is then elevated to gain access to the cortical plate [47, 49]. A cortical window is made with an osteotome or surgical drill to gain access to the cancellous component of the bone. The required cancellous bone is then harvested until the inferior component of the cortical bone is reached [49]. The wound is then closed in a layer, with the iliotibial tract approximated with resorbable sutures.

6.1 Complications

Apart from the common post-operative surgical complications like infection, wound dehiscence, pain, gait disturbance, and paraesthesia, proximal tibia fractures have seldomly been reported in the literature [2]. A study by O'Keeffe et al. of 230 patients reported only one case of fracture [50]. Hughes et al. reported 2 cases of proximal tibial fracture out of 75 cases, but these fractures were associated with alleged external injuries [51]. In a retrospective study by Ana Lucia et al. on 31 patients who underwent tibial bone harvesting, only 5 cases of minor complications were noted which all self-resolved within three weeks [52]. Kushner reported a complication rate of just 1.4% in a series of 141 patients [49]. In a meta-analysis, Shmidt et al. reported 63 complications out of 1,137 cases. Most of the complications were minor, but there were 5 cases of fracture and 1 case of osteomyelitis [48].

Despite its safety and ease, the proximal tibial harvest has not attained the same level of popularity as the iliac crest or calvarial grafts possibly as a result of unfamiliarity [47–49]. A review of the current literature nonetheless demonstrates that the tibia may be an appropriate alternative.

7. Costochondral graft

The costochondral graft was arguably the first developed autogenous graft used to reconstruct a segmental defect of the mandible. A unique advantage of rib grafts is that they can be harvested with their cartilage, active growth, and bony components, and that it may continue to grow even after application. This makes the costochondral graft a possible option for reconstruction in growing patients [53]. Anatomically, the rib's is long, curvilinear shape makes it an adequate replacement for lateral defects of the mandible involving the angle and the ramus. The cartilaginous portion can function in the temporomandibular joint even in growing individuals [54, 55]. Maxillofacial surgeons have also incorporated costochondral grafts to reconstruct the nasal dorsum and septum in cleft individuals [56, 57]. Reports of using free rib graft to reconstruct the medial and orbital floor also exist [58]. A study by Tetsuji et al. demonstrateed no significant complications after in an 8 week cohort [59].

However, the growth potential of a harvested rib is difficult to predict, as is its tendency to resorb. Literature recommends the use of relatively shorter cartilage portions (2–3 mm) [60] to limit unwanted growth [5, 61].

Relevant anatomy and surgical technique - The fifths, sixth, and seventh ribs are commonly selected for the harvesting. The cartilaginous component makes up approximately 1/3rd of the total length. An incision is placed 5 mm above the inframammary fold, and the incision is carried to the muscle level. The costochondral perichondrium lies immediately deep to the muscular fascia and must be exposed with care [2, 7, 53]. Then bony and the cartilaginous components of the ribs must be clearly identified so that the incision is placed along the longitudinal axis, and to safeguard the cartilage from any inadvertent injury [53]. The perichondrium is then reflected until the posterior aspect of the rib is exposed. Continuous palpation of the rib is essential to prevent pleural injury leading to the pneumothorax. The last step involves dividing the cartilaginous rib medially at the sternum and proximally at the bony rib [7, 53].

The graft is then shaped into the desired form by multiple osteotomies and fixated at the recipient site. Layered closure is executed at the donor site, ensuring tight closure of the perichondrium to decrease postoperative pain. A valsalva maneuver should be conducted to check for any air leakage that can lead to post-op pneumothorax. A surgical drain is usually placed to reduce the risk of pleuritis [53, 62].

7.1 Complications

Complications associated with the rib graft can be categorized into early and delayed. Early complications include pneumothorax, pleuritis, and infection; while examples of delayed complications are graft resorption and unpredictable graft growth [63, 64]. In a meta-analysis, Wee et al. studied 458 patients who underwent rhinoplasty with rib cartilage and reported 42 cases of unpredictable growth of the nasal dorsum, 4 cases of resorption, and 19 cases of hypertrophic scar formation. A systematic review by Kiran et al. reported similar findings as well [65]. A long-term study of 55 patients by Awal et al. reported that after 10 years, there were 58.9% of cases with unpredictable growth and graft resorption, 12.9% of cases with pneumothorax, and 1.8% of cases warranted immediate tracheostomy [66]. In fact, a 2015 study concluded that evidence for costochondral growth may not be sufficient. Sidebottom advises avoiding these grafts altogether due to scar tissue formation, which reduces vascular supply [67]. However, most studies stipulate that costochondral grafting is an acceptable procedure with adequate outcomes in repairing craniofacial anomalies [2, 4, 7, 53, 54, 56–59, 62, 68–70].

8. Osteointegration of NVBG

Bone healing remains unique because it relies on cellular regeneration of a calcified matrix. In NVBGs, regeneration of the graft relies entirely on recipient site vasculature, which typically initiates neo-angiogenesis starts after three days of consolidation [19, 71]. The surgeon must therefore maintain the integrity of the periosteal envelope at the recipient site as this serves as the sole nutritional source to the graft until vascularization.

There are three possible mechanisms by which bone grafts heal or integrate, and in most cases, these mechanisms work synergistically to form a new bone [19].

1. Direct osteogenesis – In direct osteogenesis, new bone forms from the surrounding periosteum and the endosteum. Surviving osteocytes within the graft play a crucial role in direct osteogenesis by recruiting new osteoblasts. Generally, the cancellous component of the bone graft heals by direct osteogenesis.

2. Osteoconduction – Here, the grafted material serves as a scaffold for the production and extension of the osseous matrix from the surrounding host bone. This matrix then serves as a conduit for additional osteoblasts and the periosteum.

3. Osteoinduction – Signaling molecules within the graft trigger osteoinduction by stimulating the osteoprogenitor cells within the surrounding host bone. Once triggered, the osteoprogenitor cells transform into osteoblasts which initiate osteogenesis. Bone morphogenic proteins are some of the most well-studied and widely utilized osteoinducing compounds in maxillofacial surgery today.

The mechanism of NVBG osteointegration remains similar irrespective of the donor site. However, the rate and amount of final bone formation differ in each case, as other factors such as recipient site integrity, nature of disease, and other patient factors also play crucial roles in final healing. In general, cortical bone heals by a method called creeping substitution [72], in which osteoclasts begin to resorb the graft material as a response to direct injury to donor's bone. These osteoclastic cells subsequently allow fibroblasts to grow and form a matrix, thereby enabling neo-vascularisation. The osteoclasts are soon occupied by osteoblastic cells from the osteoid [19, 72–74].

Further mineralization is initiated by osteoblastic cells. The synchronous activity of osteoblasts and osteoclasts forms a bone that is then remodeled prior to final maturation. The donor cortext never goes through complete resorption and remains intermixed with the new bone.

In cancellous bone, apposition precedes resorption by the ingrowth of scaffolds, on which osteoblasts form new bone [19, 74]. Structurally, cancellous bone contains marrow which allows it to revascularize rapidly. Unlike the cortices, cancellous bone undergoes complete resorption, which is then replaced by vasculature and mature bone [19, 73, 75].

Surviving osteoblasts secrete different growth factors at different periods, which expedite the healing process. Among the several growth factors, the most commonly identified ones include PDGF (plasma-derived growth factor), TGF (transforming growth factor), VEGF (vasculoendothelial growth factor), and EGF (extra-cellular growth factor). These growth factors are secreted during the second week of healing until maturation ceases [71]. Recently - with a better understanding of growth factors at the molecular level - surgeons have begun treating bone grafts with external sources of growth factor at the time of surgery. The growth factor is thought to promote healing even at the earlier stages of the graft as the host growth factors do not fully mobilize until the second week [73]. Moreover, these growth factors may promote new bone formation in the compromised recipient site which may lack healing potential as a result of devascularization or loss of embedded osteocytes.

8.1 Efficacy of craniofacial versus distal donor bone

Bone harvested from the craniofacial region usually has demonstrates lower rate of resorption than those from distant regions like the ileum, tibia, and rib. Many investigators hold that embryologic similarity in the donor and host bones allow the graft to perform better [19, 71–74, 76]. This phenomenon may be a result of the congruence of the progenitor cells and signaling factors. Others show that craniofacial bones typically contain more vascular channels, which aid in early vascularization [77, 78].

8.2 Fate of bone graft

NVBGs taken from distant sites undergo post-op resorption that typically require over-compensation of volume by approximately 20%. Animal studies using zygomatic and the iliac donor sites showed significant loss of the iliac graft and minimal loss of the zygomatic graft [18]. Preservation of the periosteum also appears to play a similar role, as intact periosteal envelopes were associated with rapid revascularization and minimal graft site volume loss [79].

9. Recent advancements in NVBG

Reconstructive surgeries have undergone significant advancements over the last few decades, both in technique and technology. Intra-operative use of platelet-rich plasma and fibrin (PRP and PRF) have shown promise in increasing graft success at minimal cost [80, 81]. In fact, leukocyte rich plasma rich fibrin (L-PRF) may stimulate osteoblastic action even more so than the traditional PRF or PRP [81]. Other biological agents like bone morphogenic protein (BMP), transforming growth factor (TGF), and insulin growth factor (IGF) have also been associated with improved success rates albeit at a higher cost [82, 83]. BMP-2 in particular has received approval from the U.S. Food and Drug Administration for its efficacy and stability [84].

Another notable advancement in the field of reconstructive surgery is intra-operative navigation. Navigation guided surgery begins by assisting surgeons in pre-operative planning and defect volume calculation in all the three planes. A spacial locator instrument is utilized intra-operatively so that the location of the instrument tip may be displayed on a rendering of the patient radiograph. With it, surgeons are able to harvest graft accurately according to the pre-operatively planned margins. Navigation also assists in ablative surgery by demonstrating the location of critical anatomical landmarks that are otherwise difficult to visualize. Surgeons can avoid nerves, arteries, and other structures without dissecting for them, reducing the risk of iatrogenic injury and subsequently the rate of graft failure [85].

10. Conclusions

NVBG remains the gold standard for managing small to mid-sized defects. Among NVBGs, the most common bone grafts used by oral and maxillofacial surgeons include the iliac crest, rib, tibia, and calvarium. With the advent of modern techniques, proximal or distal graft harvest has become a generally safe and successful component of craniofacial reconstruction.

Author details

Manish Anand* and Shreya Panwar
Meenakshi Ammal Dental College, Chennai, India

*Address all correspondence to: manishanand028@gmail.com

References

[1] Elsalanty ME, Genecov DG. Bone grafts in craniofacial surgery. Craniomaxillofacial trauma & reconstruction. 2009 Oct;2(3-4):125-34.

[2] Zouhary KJ. Bone graft harvesting from distant sites: concepts and techniques. Oral and Maxillofacial Surgery Clinics. 2010 Aug 1;22(3):301-16.

[3] Gadre PK, Ramanojam S, Patankar A, Gadre KS. Nonvascularized bone grafting for mandibular reconstruction: myth or reality?. Journal of Craniofacial Surgery. 2011 Sep 1;22(5):1727-35.

[4] Ahmed W, Asim MA, Ehsan A, Abbas Q. Non-vascularized autogenous bone grafts for reconstruction of maxillofacial osseous defects. J. Coll. Phys. Surg. Pak. 2018 Jan 1;28:17-21.

[5] Moura LB, Carvalho PD, Xavier CB, Post LK, Torriani MA, Santagata M, Júnior OC. Autogenous non-vascularized bone graft in segmental mandibular reconstruction: a systematic review. International Journal of Oral and Maxillofacial Surgery. 2016 Nov 1;45(11):1388-94.

[6] Elsalanty ME, Genecov DG. Bone grafts in craniofacial surgery. Craniomaxillofacial trauma & reconstruction. 2009 Oct;2(3-4):125-34.

[7] Ehrenfeld M, Hagenmaier C. Autogenous bone grafts in maxillofacial reconstruction. InCraniomaxillofacial reconstructive and corrective bone surgery 2019 (pp. 319-343). Springer, New York, NY.

[8] SCHMITZ JP, Hollinger JO. The critical size defect as an experimental model for craniomandibulofacial nonunions. Clinical Orthopaedics and Related Research®. 1986 Apr 1;205:299-308.

[9] Bosch C, Melsen B, Vargervik K. Importance of the critical-size bone defect in testing bone-regenerating materials. The Journal of craniofacial surgery. 1998 Jul;9(4):310-6.

[10] Hollinger JO, Kleinschmidt JC. The critical size defect as an experimental model to test bone repair materials. Journal of Craniofacial Surgery. 1990 Jan 1;1(1):60-8.

[11] Levin L, Herzberg R, Dolev E, Schwartz-Arad D. Smoking and complications of onlay bone grafts and sinus lift operations. International Journal of Oral & Maxillofacial Implants. 2004 May 1;19(3).

[12] Kawase T, Okuda K, Saito Y, Amizuka N, Suzuki H, Yoshie H. Platelet-rich plasma provides nucleus for mineralization in cultures of partially differentiated periodontal ligament cells. In Vitro Cellular & Developmental Biology-Animal. 2005 May 1;41(5-6):171-6.

[13] Okuda K, Kawase T, Momose M, Murata M, Saito Y, Suzuki H, Wolff LF, Yoshie H. Platelet-rich plasma contains high levels of platelet-derived growth factor and transforming growth factor-β and modulates the proliferation of periodontally related cells in vitro. Journal of periodontology. 2003 Jun;74(6):849-57.

[14] Bak M, Jacobson AS, Buchbinder D, Urken ML. Contemporary reconstruction of the mandible. Oral oncology. 2010 Feb 1;46(2):71-6.

[15] Allsopp BJ, Hunter-Smith DJ, Rozen WM. Vascularized versus nonvascularized bone grafts: what is the evidence?. Clinical Orthopaedics and Related Research®. 2016 May 1;474(5):1319-27.

[16] Marechek A, AlShare A, Pack S, Demko C, Quereshy FA, Baur D. Nonvascularized bone grafts for reconstruction of segmental mandibular defects: Is length of graft a factor of success?. Journal of Oral and Maxillofacial Surgery. 2019 Dec 1;77(12):2557-66.

[17] Urlaub KM, Ettinger RE, Nelson NS, Hoxie JM, Snider AE, Perosky JE, Polyatskaya Y, Donneys A, Buchman SR. Nonvascularized Bone Graft Reconstruction of the Irradiated Murine Mandible: An Analogue of Clinical Head and Neck Cancer Treatment. Journal of Craniofacial Surgery. 2019 Mar 1;30(2):611-7.

[18] Zins JE, Whitaker LA, Enlow DH. Membranous versus endochondral bone: implications for craniofacial reconstruction. Plastic and reconstructive surgery. 1983 Dec 1;72(6):785.

[19] Marx RE. Bone and bone graft healing. Oral and maxillofacial surgery clinics of North America. 2007 Nov 1;19(4):455-66.

[20] Burstein FD, Simms C, Cohen SR, Work F, Paschal M. Iliac crest bone graft harvesting techniques: a comparison. Plastic and reconstructive surgery. 2000 Jan 1;105(1):34-9.

[21] Shaw KA, Griffith MS, Shaw VM, Devine JG, Gloystein DM. Harvesting autogenous cancellous bone graft from the anterior iliac crest. JBJS Essential Surgical Techniques. 2018 Sep 28;8(3).

[22] Mischkowski RA, Selbach I, Neugebauer J, Koebke J, Zöller JE. Lateral femoral cutaneous nerve and iliac crest bone grafts—anatomical and clinical considerations. International journal of oral and maxillofacial surgery. 2006 Apr 1;35(4):366-72.

[23] Üzel M, Akkin SM, Tanyeli E, Koebke J. Relationships of the lateral femoral cutaneous nerve to bony landmarks. Clinical Orthopaedics and Related Research®. 2011 Sep 1;469(9):2605-11.

[24] Zhu JF, Xu WX, Hu Q, Wu TQ, Liu H. Iliac Bone Harvesting Techniques for Bone Reconstruction. Comparative Study Between Tricortical Bone Harvesting vs Trapdoor Technique. Therapeutics and Clinical Risk Management. 2020;16:559.

[25] Robinson BT, Metcalfe D, Cuff AV, Pidgeon TE, Hewitt KJ, Gibbs VN, Rossiter DJ, Griffin XL. Surgical techniques for autologous bone harvesting from the iliac crest in adults. The Cochrane Database of Systematic Reviews. 2018 Apr;2018(4).

[26] Robinson BT, Metcalfe D, Cuff AV, Pidgeon TE, Hewitt KJ, Gibbs VN, Rossiter DJ, Griffin XL. Surgical techniques for autologous bone harvesting from the iliac crest in adults. The Cochrane Database of Systematic Reviews. 2018 Apr;2018(4).

[27] Carson M. Anterior iliac crest bone graft. InAtlas of Operative Oral and Maxillofacial Surgery 2015 Jan 5 (pp. 475-479). Hoboken, NJ, USA: John Wiley & Sons, Inc..

[28] Ahlmann E, Patzakis M, Roidis N, Shepherd L, Holtom P. Comparison of anterior and posterior iliac crest bone grafts in terms of harvest-site morbidity and functional outcomes. JBJS. 2002 May 1;84(5):716-20.

[29] Morrissey PB, Nadeau RA, Hoffmeister EP. Posterior Iliac Crest Bone Graft. Atlas of Operative Oral and Maxillofacial Surgery. 2015 Jan 9:54.

[30] Abramowicz S, Katsnelson A, Forbes PW, Padwa BL. Anterior versus posterior approach to iliac crest for alveolar cleft bone grafting. Journal of oral and maxillofacial surgery. 2012 Jan 1;70(1):211-5.

[31] Kolomvos N, Iatrou I, Theologie-Lygidakis N, Tzerbos F, Schoinohoriti O. Iliac crest morbidity following maxillofacial bone grafting in children: a clinical and radiographic prospective study. Journal of Cranio-Maxillofacial Surgery. 2010 Jun 1;38(4):293-302.

[32] Cricchio G, Lundgren S. Donor site morbidity in two different approaches to anterior iliac crest bone harvesting. Clinical implant dentistry and related research. 2003 Oct;5(3):161-9.

[33] Barone A, Ricci M, Mangano F, Covani U. Morbidity associated with iliac crest harvesting in the treatment of maxillary and mandibular atrophies: a 10-year analysis. Journal of oral and maxillofacial surgery. 2011 Sep 1;69(9):2298-304.

[34] Almaiman M, Al-Bargi HH, Manson P. Complication of anterior iliac bone graft harvesting in 372 adult patients from May 2006 to May 2011 and a literature review. Craniomaxillofacial trauma & reconstruction. 2013 Dec;6(4):257-65.

[35] Fasolis M, Boffano P, Ramieri G. Morbidity associated with anterior iliac crest bone graft. Oral surgery, oral medicine, oral pathology and oral radiology. 2012 Nov 1;114(5):586-91.

[36] Mazock JB, Schow SR, Triplett RG. Posterior iliac crest bone harvest: review of technique, complications, and use of an epidural catheter for postoperative pain control1. Journal of oral and maxillofacial surgery. 2003 Dec 1;61(12):1497-503.

[37] Nkenke E, Weisbach V, Winckler E, Kessler P, Schultze-Mosgau S, Wiltfang J, Neukam FW. Morbidity of harvesting of bone grafts from the iliac crest for preprosthetic augmentation procedures: a prospective study. International journal of oral and maxillofacial surgery. 2004 Mar 1;33(2):157-63.

[38] Frodel JL, Marentette LJ, Quatela VC, Weinstein GS. Calvarial bone graft harvest: Techniques, considerations, and morbidity. Archives of Otolaryngology–Head & Neck Surgery. 1993 Jan 1;119(1):17-23.

[39] Kline JR, Wolfe SA. Complications associated with the harvesting of cranial bone grafts. Plastic and reconstructive surgery. 1995 Jan;95(1):5-13.

[40] Cheney ML, Gliklich RE. The use of calvarial bone in nasal reconstruction. Archives of Otolaryngology–Head & Neck Surgery. 1995 Jun 1;121(6):643-8.

[41] Harsha BC, Turvey TA, Powers SK. Use of autogenous cranial bone grafts in maxillofacial surgery: a preliminary report. Journal of oral and maxillofacial surgery. 1986 Jan 1;44(1):11-5.

[42] Agrawal A, Garg LN. Split calvarial bone graft for the reconstruction of skull defects. Journal of surgical technique and case report. 2011 Jan;3(1):13.

[43] Maves MD, Matt BH. Calvarial bone grafting of facial defects. Otolaryngology—Head and Neck Surgery. 1986 Nov;95(4):464-70.

[44] Casanova R, Cavalcante D, Grotting JC, Vasconez LO, Psillakis JM. Anatomic basis for vascularized outer-table calvarial bone flaps. Plastic and reconstructive surgery. 1986 Sep 1;78(3):300-8.

[45] Touzet S, Ferri J, Wojcik T, Raoul G. Complications of calvarial bone harvesting for maxillofacial reconstructions. Journal of Craniofacial Surgery. 2011 Jan 1;22(1):178-81.

[46] Aydin S, Kucukyuruk B, Abuzayed B, Aydin S, Sanus GZ. Cranioplasty: review of materials and techniques. Journal of neurosciences in rural practice. 2011 Jul;2(2):162.

[47] Ko EC, Chang CM, Chang P, Kao CC, Chen KJ, Wu IF, Chen MY. Tibial Cancellous Bone Grafting in Jaw Reconstruction: 10 Years of Experience in Taiwan. Clinical implant dentistry and related research. 2015 Jan;17:e321-31.

[48] Schmidt ER, Townsend J. Unusual complication of subacute osteomyelitis following tibial bone graft: report of a case. Journal of oral and maxillofacial surgery. 2008 Jun 1;66(6):1290-3.

[49] Kushner GM. Tibia bone graft harvest technique. Atlas of the oral and maxillofacial surgery clinics of North America. 2005 Sep 1;13(2):119-26.

[50] Engelstad ME, Morse T. Anterior iliac crest, posterior iliac crest, and proximal tibia donor sites: a comparison of cancellous bone volumes in fresh cadavers. Journal of oral and maxillofacial surgery. 2010 Dec 1;68(12):3015-21.

[51] Hughes CW, Revington PJ. The proximal tibia donor site in cleft alveolar bone grafting: experience of 75 consecutive cases. Journal of Cranio-Maxillofacial Surgery. 2002 Feb 1;30(1):12-6.

[52] Miceli AL, Pereira LC, da Silva Torres T, Calasans-Maia M, Louro RS. Mandibular reconstruction with lateral tibial bone graft: an excellent option for oral and maxillofacial surgery. Craniomaxillofacial Trauma & Reconstruction. 2017 Dec;10(4):292-8.

[53] Abdel-Haleem AK, Nouby R, Taghian M. The use of the rib grafts in head and neck reconstruction. Egyptian Journal of Ear, Nose, Throat and Allied Sciences. 2011 Jul 1;12(2):89-98.

[54] Fernandes R, Fattahi T, Steinberg B. Costochondral rib grafts in mandibular reconstruction. Atlas of the oral and maxillofacial surgery clinics of North America. 2006 Sep 1;14(2):179-83.

[55] Poswillo D. Experimental reconstruction of the mandibular joint. International journal of oral surgery. 1974 Jan 1;3(6):400-11.

[56] Moretti A, Sciuto S. Rib grafts in septorhinoplasty. Acta Otorhinolaryngologica Italica. 2013 Jun;33(3):190.

[57] Daniel RK. Rhinoplasty and rib grafts: evolving a flexible operative technique. Plastic and reconstructive surgery. 1994 Oct 1;94(5):597-609.

[58] Johnson PE, Raftopoulos I. In situ splitting of a rib graft for reconstruction of the orbital floor. Plastic and reconstructive surgery. 1999 May 1;103(6):1709-11.

[59] Uemura T, Yanai T, Yasuta M, Harada Y, Morikawa A, Watanabe H, Kurokawa M. In Situ Splitting of a Rib Bone Graft for Reconstruction of Orbital Floor and Medial Wall. Craniomaxillofacial trauma & reconstruction. 2017 Jun;10(2):123-9.

[60] Khadka A, Hu J. Autogenous grafts for condylar reconstruction in treatment of TMJ ankylosis: current concepts and considerations for the future. International journal of oral and maxillofacial surgery. 2012 Jan 1;41(1):94-102.

[61] Guyuron B, Lasa Jr CI. Unpredictable growth pattern of costochondral graft. Plastic and reconstructive surgery. 1992 Nov 1;90(5):880-6.

[62] Christophel JJ, Hilger PA. Osseocartilaginous rib graft rhinoplasty: a stable, predictable technique for major dorsal reconstruction. Archives of Facial Plastic Surgery. 2011 Mar 21;13(2):78-83.

[63] Wee JH, Park MH, Oh S, Jin HR. Complications associated with autologous rib cartilage use in rhinoplasty: a meta-analysis. JAMA

facial plastic surgery. 2015 Jan 1;17(1):49-55.

[64] Kumar P, Rattan V, Rai S. Do costochondral grafts have any growth potential in temporomandibular joint surgery? A systematic review. Journal of oral biology and craniofacial research. 2015 Sep 1;5(3):198-202.

[65] Varadharajan K, Sethukumar P, Anwar M, Patel K. Complications associated with the use of autologous costal cartilage in rhinoplasty: a systematic review. Aesthetic surgery journal. 2015 Aug 1;35(6):644-52.

[66] Awal DH, Jaffer M, Charan G, Ball RE, Kennedy G, Thomas S, Farook SA, Mills C, Ayliffe P. Costochondral grafting for paediatric temporomandibular joint reconstruction: 10-year outcomes in 55 cases. International Journal of Oral and Maxillofacial Surgery. 2018 Nov 1;47(11):1433-8.

[67] Sidebottom AJ. Alloplastic or autogenous reconstruction of the TMJ. journal of oral biology and craniofacial research. 2013 Sep 1;3(3):135-9.

[68] Caccamese JF, Ruiz RL, Costello BJ. Costochondral rib grafting. Atlas of the oral and maxillofacial surgery clinics of North America. 2005 Sep 1;13(2):139-49.

[69] Sharma H, Chowdhury S, Navaneetham A, Upadhyay S, Alam S. Costochondral graft as interpositional material for TMJ ankylosis in children: a clinical study. Journal of maxillofacial and oral surgery. 2015 Sep 1;14(3):565-72.

[70] Sahoo NK, Tomar K, Kumar A, Roy ID. Selecting reconstruction option for TMJ ankylosis: a surgeon's dilemma. Journal of Craniofacial Surgery. 2012 Nov 1;23(6):1796-801..

[71] Cypher TJ, Grossman JP. Biological principles of bone graft healing. The Journal of foot and ankle surgery. 1996 Sep 1;35(5):413-7.

[72] Kalfas IH. Principles of bone healing. Neurosurgical focus. 2001 Apr 1;10(4):1-4.

[73] Bartlett SP, Whitaker LA. Growth and survival of vascularized and nonvascularized membranous bone: An experimental study. Plastic and reconstructive surgery. 1989 Nov 1;84(5):783-8.

[74] LaTrenta GS, McCarthy JG, Cutting CB. The growth of vascularized onlay bone transfers. Annals of plastic surgery. 1987 Jun;18(6):511-6.

[75] Smith JD, Abramson M. Membranous vs endochondral bone autografts. Archives of Otolaryngology. 1974 Mar 1;99(3):203-5.

[76] Kusiak JF, Zins JE, Whitaker LA. The early revascularization of membranous bone. Plastic and reconstructive surgery. 1985 Oct 1;76(4):510-4.

[77] THOMPSON N, CASSON JA. Experimental onlay bone grafts to the jaws: a preliminary study in dogs. Plastic and reconstructive surgery. 1970 Oct 1;46(4):341-9.

[78] KNIZE DM. THE INFLUENCE OF PERIOSTEUM AND CALCTTONIN ON ONLAY BONE GRAFT SURVIVAL A Roentgenographic Study. Plastic and Reconstructive Surgery. 1974 Feb 1;53(2):190-9.

[79] Alberius MG. Some basic factors essential to autogeneic nonvascularized onlay bone grafting to the craniofacial skeleton. Scandinavian journal of plastic and reconstructive surgery and hand surgery. 1999 Jan 1;33(2):129-46.

[80] Del Corso M, Vervelle A, Simonpieri A, Jimbo R, Inchingolo F, Sammartino G, M Dohan Ehrenfest D. Current knowledge and perspectives

for the use of platelet-rich plasma (PRP) and platelet-rich fibrin (PRF) in oral and maxillofacial surgery part 1: Periodontal and dentoalveolar surgery. Current Pharmaceutical Biotechnology. 2012 Jun 1;13(7):1207-30.

[81] Simonpieri A, Del Corso M, Vervelle A, Jimbo R, Inchingolo F, Sammartino G, M Dohan Ehrenfest D. Current knowledge and perspectives for the use of platelet-rich plasma (PRP) and platelet-rich fibrin (PRF) in oral and maxillofacial surgery part 2: Bone graft, implant and reconstructive surgery. Current Pharmaceutical Biotechnology. 2012 Jun 1;13(7):1231-56.

[82] Janicki P, Schmidmaier G. What should be the characteristics of the ideal bone graft substitute? Combining scaffolds with growth factors and/or stem cells. Injury. 2011 Sep 1;42:S77-81.

[83] Simpson AH, Mills L, Noble B. The role of growth factors and related agents in accelerating fracture healing. The Journal of bone and joint surgery. British volume. 2006 Jun;88(6):701-5.

[84] Schliephake H. Bone growth factors in maxillofacial skeletal reconstruction. International journal of oral and maxillofacial surgery. 2002 Oct 1;31(5):469-84.

[85] Feichtinger M, Zemann W, Mossböck R, Kärcher H. Three-dimensional evaluation of secondary alveolar bone grafting using a 3D-navigation system based on computed tomography: a two-year follow-up. British Journal of Oral and Maxillofacial Surgery. 2008 Jun 1;46(4):278-82.

Section 3

Surgical and Anesthetic Airway Techniques

Chapter 5

Principles of Anesthesia and Airway Management in Head and Neck Surgery

Muhammad Jaffar Khan, Tarek Tageldin, Muhammad Waqas Farooqi, Odai Qasim Khamash, Umair Shahid, Mohamed El-Fatih Abdul-Rahman, Mohamed Elarref and Jazib Hassan

Abstract

This topic aims to discuss key aspects of anesthetic and airway management for head and neck surgery. Airway management is a central part of patient care and management in Head and Neck Surgery. Common challenges in Head and Neck surgery are shared airway, distorted airway anatomy due to existing pathology; risk of airway obstruction, disconnection or loss of airway intra-operatively; risk of soiling of the airway due to bleeding and surgical debris; and the potential for airway compromise post-operatively. The option for airway management technique is influenced by patient's factors, anesthetic needs, and surgical requirements. Intubation technique necessitating either a small or large cuffed tracheal tube with a throat pack provides the highest level of airway protection Non-intubation or open airway techniques involve mask ventilation, apneic techniques, and insufflation techniques, or the use of a laryngeal mask airway. Lastly, jet ventilation techniques may be conducted via a supraglottic, subglottic or transtracheal routes. It is essential to have clear airway management plans including rescue airway strategies that should be communicated with the surgeons and patients at the earliest opportunity.

Keywords: head and neck surgery, shared airway, airway management, anesthesia management, preoperative endoscopy, total intravenous anesthesia (TIVA), bronchoscopy, transoral robotic surgery, functional endoscopic surgery, laser surgery, virtual endoscopy

1. Introduction

Head and neck (H&N) surgery encompasses an expanded spectrum of procedures varying greatly in complexity, duration, and complications. They range from simple surgeries such as dental procedure, adenotonsillectomy to precise and image-guided laryngologic, neurotologic, and skull-base surgery, complex obstructive sleep apnea (OSA) surgery, sophisticated transoral robotic surgery (TORS), transoral laser microsurgery (TLM), and major head and neck oncological surgery with extensive free-flap reconstruction.

Head and neck surgery presents unprecedented challenges for the anesthesiologists including shared airways, concurrent comorbidities, anesthesia techniques, and postoperative complications. A Shared Airway is the term commonly used in Head and Neck surgery which is characterized by "any procedure where the anesthesiologist needs to maintain a patient's airway patency, oxygenation, and ventilation in a similar airway anatomical space in which the surgeon operates." Both the anesthetists and surgeons must have a clear knowledge and understanding of their respective roles in managing the 'shared airway'. The role of the anesthetist must be to provide safe general anesthesia for the patient, an uninterrupted airway during the perioperative period, and a clear field for the surgeon by applying various hypotensive anesthesia techniques. This chapter focuses on key aspects of anesthesia and airway management strategies for common Head and Neck surgical presentations, with relevance to the current evidence base and clinical guidelines. It is aimed to be a comprehensive review for residents and fellows training in the fields of anesthesia and head and neck surgery.

2. Difficult airway management in head and neck (H&N) surgery: background

It is estimated that the occurrence of difficult airway and complications are more frequent in H&N patients than in the general surgical population. In the Fourth National Audit Project (NAP4) from the Royal College of Anesthetists and the Difficult Airway Society in the United Kingdom (UK), data regarding major airway complications were collected prospectively in approximately three million anesthetized patients throughout the UK [1]. The incidence of airway-related complications was nearly 40% in H&N surgeries [2] and almost 75% of the cases required emergency surgical airway (ESA) for "cannot intubate/cannot oxygenate" (CICO) situations. Likewise, the incidence of the emergency surgical airway (ESA) was even higher in another retrospective study of 452,461 patients in the Danish Anesthesia Database [3]. In this study, the overall incidence of ESA in ear, nose, and throat surgery was reported as 1.6 events per thousand, which was 27 times higher than in the general surgical population (0.06 per thousand). The H&N oncological patients are at even higher risk of difficult airway management, predominantly males, with an incidence of over 12% experienced difficult direct laryngoscopy and tracheal intubation [4]. In NAP4, of the 21 cases of difficult

Factors associated with airway management related complication	Inadequate airway assessment
	Inadequate planning for airway management and for failure of intubation
	Multiple intubation attempts
	Inappropriate use of a supraglottic airway (SGA) device
	Obesity
	Failure to correctly interpret capnography and recognize esophageal intubation early
	Anesthesia for head and neck surgery
	Intubation in the emergency department or intensive care unit

Table 1.
NAP4 identified several factors associated with major airway complications.

airway observed on anesthesia induction, 13 cases occurred in patients with upper airway tumors [1]. Additionally, numerous studies have indicated that difficult tracheal intubation, defined as three or more attempts on direct laryngoscopy, may be observed in up to 7–9% of H&N cases [5–7], which is up to four folds higher than the general surgical population [8–11]. In the NAP4 study, several factors have been associated with airway related complications (see **Table 1**). Furthermore, anesthesiologists experience greater challenges during extubation and post-anesthesia recovery period [1, 12].

3. General principles: preoperative assessment

The preoperative Anesthesia assessment is imperative in reducing risk during shared airway procedure and must include a detailed general medical and surgical history, previous anesthetic exposure, and general physical examination as well as a focused airway assessment. It is paramount to have a multidisciplinary approach to an anticipated difficult airway in H&N surgery which requires a high degree of cooperation and communication with the surgeon, allowing for early identification of high-risk patients, and reciprocal anticipation of the potential problems and adequate preparation to face the challenges. Expertise in H&N anesthesia and complex airway management should be encouraged as it improves the outcome and reduces airway complications. The goal of preoperative assessment is to recognize patients with potentially difficult airways, stratify the risks, manage the co-morbidities, and optimize the patient's condition before major H&N surgery (see **Table 2**).

3.1 Airway assessment: history and physical exam

Preanesthesia assessment invariably includes airway evaluation to identify and predict difficulty in airway management. The incidence of difficult airway is higher for patients who undergo H&N surgeries than for general surgical procedures. Therefore, the primary priority in airway assessment is to determine whether airway is compromised. A detailed history should be obtained before the surgery which incorporates reviewing previous anesthesia records with a particular focus on airway management, identifying risk factors of possible difficult mask ventilation and tracheal intubation. History of previous difficult tracheal intubation is one of the most important predictors of the anticipated difficult airway [9, 11]. It is worth mentioning that a history of prior easy intubation does not guarantee

Anesthesia considerations in Head and Neck Surgery	Multidisciplinary approach and close-in line communication
	Presence of expertise in H&N anesthesia and complex airway management
	Anticipation of challenges during intubation and extubation
	Shared Airway with the surgeon and related challenges
	Different approach to airway management specific to surgery
	Different Anesthesia technique and positioning challenges
	Post Anesthesia recovery and Airway support

Table 2.
Anesthesia considerations in head and neck surgery.

subsequent uneventful airway management in H&N procedures, due to the progression of the underlying pathological processes and their significant effect on the airway anatomy [13]. Anatomic anomaly relating to the face, mouth, nose, pharynx, or larynx must be thoroughly investigated. Hoarseness, drooling, dysphagia, orthopnea, stridor, cough, and recent onset of snoring may indicate airway compromise. Patients with vocal cord paralysis may be at increased risk for perioperative pulmonary aspiration. Prior H&N radiotherapy induces tissue fibrosis as well as long-standing epiglottic and glottic edema, leading to a non-compliant airway with limited mouth opening and restricted neck movement [9], which may make both mask ventilation and laryngoscopy potentially difficult [14]. Routine bedside airway assessment tools can be performed such as the American Society of Anesthesiologists (ASA) bedside airway assessment tool which includes Mallampati classification, thyromental distance, inter-incisor distance, neck mobility, and body mass index (BMI), etc. [15]. However, it is poorly predictive of difficult airway in Head and Neck surgery because it fails to assess the inside pathology and severity of the upper airway such as base of the tongue, glottic and vallecular lesions, etc. [8, 16]. Numerous risk factors associated with difficult airway management have been identified (see **Table 3**) [17].

3.2 Pre-operative assessment of comorbidities

Head and Neck surgery may entail a wide range of patient populations from young and healthy to elderly, geriatric patients with significant cardiovascular, respiratory, endocrine, and renal diseases who are also at high risk for postoperative delirium and cognitive dysfunction. The perioperative risk related to major H&N surgery rises with advanced age and an increased number of comorbidities. As part of the multidisciplinary team, the anesthesiologist plays a crucial role in deciding the treatment plans, optimizing the patient's condition pre-operatively, and weighing the risk to benefit ratio of the surgery. Patients with cardiovascular diseases such as uncontrolled hypertension, cerebrovascular, and coronary artery disease, chronic renal insufficiency, must be evaluated for cardiac risk prior to noncardiac surgery and if required must be referred to cardiologists. Cardiopulmonary exercise testing (CPET) can be a useful aid to decision making, particularly where more extensive or complex surgery is being performed. Also, poorly controlled heart failure (New York Heart Association Grade 3–4) is associated with poor prognosis. Brain natriuretic peptide (BNP) and N-terminal proBNP are useful biomarkers for

Risk factors for predicted difficult airway management	Mallampati grade 3 or 4
	Decreased thyromental distance
	Male gender and Age > 57 years
	Absence of teeth
	Presence of beard
	Obstructive sleep apnea or History of snoring
	Dencreased Mandibular protrusion
	Thick or short neck
	Neck radiation changes or a neck mass
	Obesity (BMI > 30)

Table 3.
Risk factors associated with difficult airway management [17].

perioperative screening of heart failure patients. Moreover, the hypotensive anesthesia technique should be avoided and intraoperative hyper or hypotension should be aggressively managed. Pulmonary comorbidities are common in H&N patients. Preoperative optimization of Chronic obstructive pulmonary disease (COPD) via treatment of acute infection and appropriate use of bronchodilators and steroids is crucial to prevent post-operative pulmonary complications. Furthermore, COPD patients may not tolerate intraoperative ventilation techniques such as spontaneous ventilation, one-lung ventilation, apneic intermittent, or jet ventilation. Likewise, patients with obstructive sleep apnea (OSA) are predisposed to difficult or challenging airways and are more sensitive to sedatives and opioids which should be used cautiously. H&N procedures involving the lower cranial nerves (Cranial nerves X, XI, and XII) may increase the risk of airway obstruction or aspiration in the post-operative period. H&N cancer patients are of particular concern as smoking and alcohol are the common cause of cancer, which also predispose them to post-operative malnutrition.

3.3 Pre-operative investigations and imaging studies

Head and Neck surgery patients must have baseline investigations which include complete blood count, biochemical profile with urea and electrolytes, coagulation profile, liver function test, blood sugar, and electrocardiography. Other investigations such as chest x-ray, pulmonary function tests, and arterial blood gases may be requested based on the risk factors and symptoms at presentation.

Imaging studies with computed tomography (CT) or magnetic resonance imaging (MRI) and flexible nasal endoscopy aid to determine the extent of the pathology and its impact on the airway and the surrounding soft tissues. The preoperative endoscopic airway examination (PEAE) in particular is useful for examining the upper airway to assess the significance of the swelling and distortion, the location, size, the spread of the lesions, the degree of obstruction, and vocal cords' mobility. Moreover, preoperative awake nasal endoscopy can be carried out by the anesthesiologist before induction which gives a real-time image of the upper airway and the larynx and is useful in formulating airway management strategies including awake intubation and surgical airway [18].

3.4 Premedication

Premedication to reduce anxiety and secretions may be helpful in patients going for H&N surgery with minor airway lesions but should be avoided in patients with H&N masses compromising the airway. Antisialagogues may be administered in the preoperative phase to minimize oral and tracheobronchial secretions. The patient should be monitored closely when premedicated, preferably in the holding area of the OR. During the preoperative visit, anesthesiologist should attempt to reduce the patient's fears and anxiety.

4. Intraoperative anesthesia management of H&N surgery

The main intraoperative goal is the appropriate choice of airway technique and airway device tailored to the patient and surgical technique. Other goals are the provision of expert airway management, a continuous plane of anesthesia, clear and immobility of the surgical field, smooth and fast recovery from anesthesia. and surgery with the implementation of enhanced recovery after surgery (ERAS) protocol for fast-track discharge of patients [19].

4.1 Anesthesia management

4.1.1 Intraoperative monitoring technique

Standard American Society of Anesthesiologists (ASA) monitors [20] such as Blood pressure, Electrocardiography, Pulse oximetry for O2 saturation, capnography, and temperature monitoring are usually applied during H&N surgery. Invasive blood pressure monitoring and advanced hemodynamic monitoring is usually considered in patients with significant cardiovascular disease or long procedures, and when excessive blood loss is expected. One study suggested that the use of goal-directed fluid therapy based on cardiac output monitoring helps guide fluid therapy and avoid fluid overload in free flap transfer [21]. Processed electroencephalogram (EEG) monitoring helps assess the depth of anesthesia and guide anesthetic drug dosing to provide a stable plane of anesthesia during surgery. Moreover, Neuromonitoring such as electromyography (EMG) monitoring of facial nerve in some head and neck surgery may guide to modify the anesthesia technique accordingly.

4.1.2 Positioning

The majority of head and neck surgeries are done in a supine position with a 15–20-degree head-up tilt to improve venous drainage. Anesthesiologists must pay meticulous attention to the patient's positioning especially since the head of the operating table is usually turned 90–180 degrees away from the anesthesia machine, limiting immediate access to the airway. Thus, long ventilator tubing and vascular access lines are required and the endotracheal tube should be secured effectively to avoid accidental extubation and disconnection. The eyes should be protected with an occlusive dressing to keep the lid closed and to prevent skin preparation solution from entering the eyes. Goggles or eye pads may be used; all pressure points must be padded, and intermittent pneumatic calf compression is applied.

4.1.3 Fluid management and blood loss

Large-bore venous access is essential for major resections when significant blood loss is anticipated. Also, the need for invasive or advanced cardiac output monitoring is determined by the patient's comorbidities as well as the nature and extent of the surgery. They are useful in assessing fluid response and guiding fluid therapy. Hypotensive anesthesia and hemodilution techniques may minimize blood loss, but must be practiced with care to maintain adequate blood flow to free flaps. Moreover, urine output should be monitored in prolonged surgeries.

4.1.4 Choice of anesthesia techniques

General anesthesia is the technique of choice as it provides airway protection, ensures adequate oxygenation, ventilation, immobility, and avoids distracting the surgeon. In some selected H&N surgeries, monitored anesthesia care can be provided to maintain spontaneous ventilation and a responsive patient with intact airway reflexes. The choice of induction technique for general anesthesia (intravenous versus inhalational agents) is based on patient factors, surgical needs, and potential for compromised ventilation. Preoperative assessment and consultation with the surgeon will determine the technique of endotracheal intubation (awake or asleep), selection of an intravenous versus inhalation induction technique, and whether to use a neuromuscular blocking agent (usually avoided if

Advantages of TIVA in Head and Neck surgery	Rapid titration of anesthesia to the desired clinical effect
	Allows immobility and facilitates nerve monitoring
	Allows rapid and smooth emergence after surgery
	Reduction in Postoperative Nausea and vomiting
	Induction of moderate hypotension may reduce blood loss and provide clear surgical field
	Technique of choice in laryngologic surgery during jet ventilation or intermittent apnea ventilation

Table 4.
Advantages of Total intravenous anesthesia in head and neck surgery.

nerve monitoring to be used intraoperatively). The NAP4 report highlighted that inhalation induction may result in total airway obstruction in patients with H&N pathology, where patients do not exhale the anesthetic gases and rapid hypoxia ensues. The theoretical advantage of gas induction is that it is a slow induction that preserves spontaneous ventilation. Additionally, maintenance of anesthesia can be obtained either with total intravenous anesthesia (TIVA) or inhalation anesthetics or a combination of inhalation anesthetic with intravenous infusion of a short-acting anesthetic. Because many H&N surgeries are associated with high incidences of postoperative nausea and vomiting (PONV), propofol-based anesthesia may be a preferable technique of choice to prevent PONV [19, 22]. Many centers use total intravenous anesthesia (TIVA) with target-controlled infusion (TCI) of propofol and opioids (see **Table 4**). In TCI, pumps are programmed to deliver an induction bolus followed by a maintenance infusion based on patient's demographics. TIVA is also useful to facilitate a clear surgical field by titrating the anesthetics to desired blood pressure [systolic blood pressure below 100 mmHg and mean arterial pressure of 60 to 70 mmHg [23]]. However, controlled hypotension should be avoided in patients with uncontrolled blood pressure, cerebrovascular or coronary artery disease, as well as chronic renal and hepatic insufficiency.

4.2 Preparing and planning for airway management

Devising safe and optimal airway management depends on close in line communication between the anesthesiologist and surgeon, airway evaluation, reviewing imaging studies, type of surgery, location of the lesion, patient's symptoms, and tolerance of the procedure and knowing the risk associated.

4.3 Airway management techniques

The technique for airway management should be formulated with the surgeon preoperatively which includes reviewing preoperative imaging studies and endoscopy, choice of airway management device, route for tracheal intubation, awake versus sleep endotracheal intubation, use of jet ventilation, and backup strategies, including preparation for a surgical airway. The goal of a pre-planned and optimal airway approach is to achieve adequate ventilation, oxygenation, and airway protection against aspiration. The following general airway management strategies should be considered:

- General anesthesia with endotracheal intubation
- General anesthesia using a supraglottic device

- General anesthesia using an Operative laryngoscopy in conjunction with jet ventilation
- Use of intermittent apnea
- General anesthesia using the patient's natural airway or spontaneous ventilation
- Local anesthesia in conjunction with intravenous sedation, with the patient breathing spontaneously

4.3.1 Options for endotracheal intubation technique

4.3.1.1 Laryngoscopy technique

It is often prudent to opt for video-laryngoscopy (VL) as a primary tracheal intubation technique because most H&N patients have high incidences of anticipated difficult airway. Multiple attempts with direct laryngoscopy (DL) should be avoided as it will lead to bleeding, soiling, edema, and fragmentation of any friable tissue in the airway that may dramatically worsen the subsequent laryngoscopic view and facemask ventilation [1, 24]. Thus, VL could be considered as a primary intubation technique in H&N patients to maximize the likelihood of first-attempt success [25]. In one meta-analysis of randomized controlled trials that compared VL versus DL in patients with anticipated or simulated difficult airways, VL was associated with improved glottic view, more likely successful intubation, and a higher chance of first-attempt intubations [26]. The provider should nonetheless approach all anticipated difficulties with caution. In one study, there was an overlap in predictive factors such as previous radiotherapy, malignancy, and previous surgery that led to difficulty in both DL and VL [27].

In conclusion, multiple attempts should be avoided as it leads to airway trauma and obstruction and alternative laryngoscopic or intubation techniques should be considered with caution (**Figures 1** and **2**).

4.3.1.2 Comparison between awake and asleep flexible fiberoptic endotracheal intubation in head and neck surgery

There is a common perception that awake fiberoptic intubation (AFOI) is the safest approach to difficult airway management [28]. Certainly, advantages of maintenance of airway patency, gas exchange, and protection against aspiration during the intubation process are offered by awake intubation. AFOI is helpful in patients with supraglottic obstruction, e.g. epiglottic or tongue base obstruction, but it is not the preferred technique in patients with a critically narrowed laryngeal inlet where there are copious secretions, difficulty in maintenance of spontaneous ventilation, and small laryngeal aperture. Adequate topicalization is key to the patient's comfort and successful airway management. Asleep fiberoptic intubation has certain benefits such as patient comfort, avoidance of anxiety, and smooth transformation to other airway devices if necessary. However, asleep fiber optic intubation may lead to a difficult airway due to airway collapse and hypoxia from depressed respiratory function. The possibility of a successful exit strategy must be evaluated when considering asleep fiber optic intubation. In NAP4, both awake and asleep flexible fiberoptic intubation have relatively high failure rates in patients with H&N pathology, with a frequency up to 60 percent [1, 29]. The most common causes for failure of flexible scope intubation include the inability to identify the

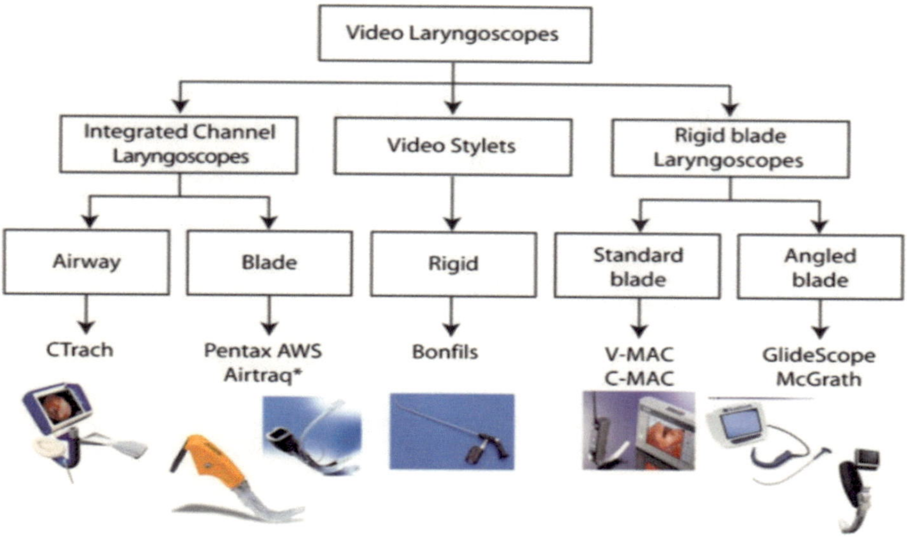

Figure 1.
A classification of video laryngoscopic devices. CTrach image courtesy of LMA North America. Pentax AWS image courtesy of Ambu USA. Airtraq image courtesy of Prodol Meditec S.A. Bonfils and C-MACA ^ VC 2012 Photo Courtesy of KARL STORZ Endoscopy-America, Inc. GlideScope image courtesy of Verathon, USA. The McGrath series 5 image courtesy of Aircraft Medical, UK. VC 2012 Healy et al.; licensee BioMed Central Ltd. Reproduced under the terms of its Creative Commons Attribution License (2.0).

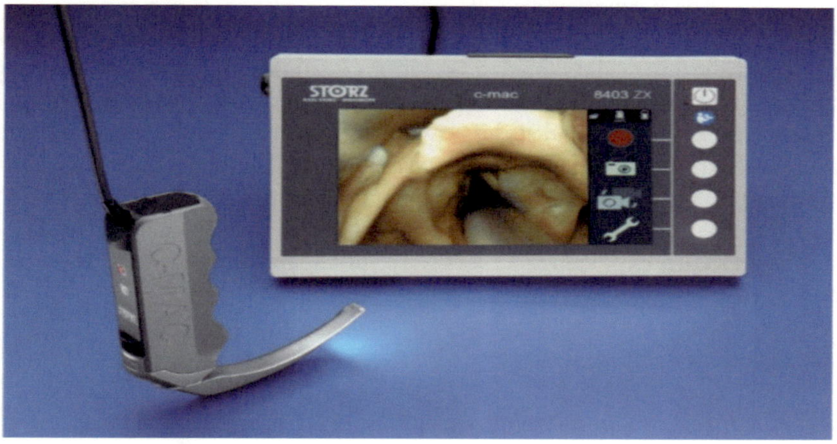

Figure 2.
4th generation Video Laryngoscope.jpg" by KARL STORZ Endoscope is licensed with CC BY-SA 4.0. To view a copy of this license, visit https://creativecommons.org/licenses/by-sa/4.0.

glottis, difficulty passing the scope, bleeding, and airway obstruction. In conclusion, awake fiberoptic intubation should be considered first in patients with head and neck pathology with an understanding of the pre-existing limitations to flexible scope intubation.

4.3.1.3 Surgical laryngoscopy and rigid bronchoscopy

Rescue endotracheal intubation using operative laryngoscopy such as anterior commissure scope or rigid bronchoscope (**Figure 3**) has been effective and shown to be successful in difficult airway scenarios or when direct laryngoscopy fails [31–33]. Hillel and colleagues have shown that the use of surgical laryngoscopes helped secure over 35% of difficult airways and reduced the number of emergent

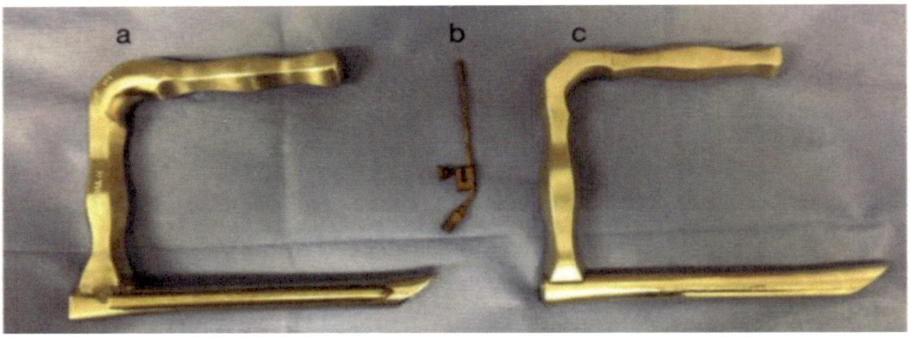

Figure 3.
ENT endoscope examples. (a) Dedo scope with external channel for light source; (b) Venturi jet for insertion into rigid scope; and (c) anterior commissure scope with narrower lumen. Reprinted from [30] Published by Elsevier Ltd.

cricothyroidotomies to nearly half [34]. After an operative laryngoscope or rigid bronchoscope is placed, manual ventilation can be provided safely through the lumen of the scope and subsequently, endotracheal intubation can be performed with the aid of an airway exchange catheter or a gum elastic bougie [35]. Thus, operative laryngoscopy and rigid bronchoscopy can rescue failed tracheal intubation and cannot intubate/cannot oxygenate (CICO) situations.

4.3.1.4 Optical stylet intubation devices

Optical intubation stylets (such as Bonfils, Clarus video System, Sensascope, Levitan optical stylets, etc.) may be helpful and offer an advantage over flexible scopes. These rigid optical stylets can help bypass mobile supraglottic and glottic masses, and once the glottis is entered, the endotracheal tube will follow the trajectory of the stylet in the patient's trachea. However, studies reported a wide range of success rates with the use of optical stylet [36, 37]. Success rates are higher with experienced users with the mean time to intubation at 23 seconds [38].

4.3.2 Supraglottic airway devices

Laryngeal mask airway (LMA) devices (**Figure 4**) offer many advantages in H&N surgery. They may be used:

- as primary ventilator devices and to provide smooth emergence from anesthesia in many elective H&N surgeries, such as ear, nasal and intranasal surgery, and facial cosmetic surgery.

- as conduits for endotracheal intubation (intubating LMA).

- as rescue devices in patients who are difficult to intubate or mask ventilate.

If LMAs are deemed necessary, the anesthetist should opt for the second generation whose seal design have been shown with less leakage and reduced risk of aspiration.

However, there are limitations to the supraglottic airway devices in H&N pathology. They may be difficult to place in patients with history of neck irradiation; limited mouth opening; and glottic, hypopharyngeal, or subglottic lesions.

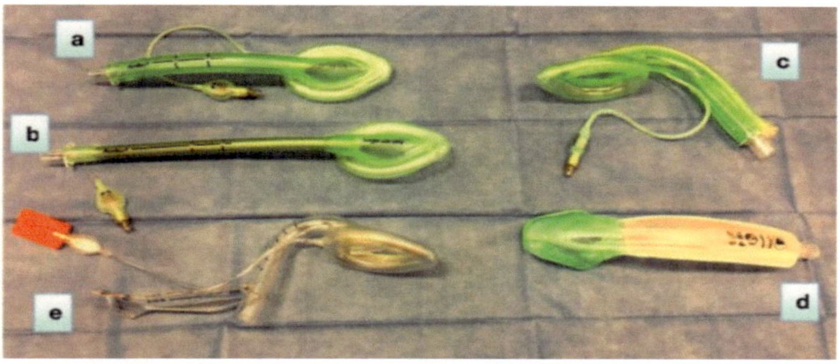

Figure 4.
Supraglottic airway devices (single use). (a) Classic LMA (Ambu AuraStraight disposable laryngeal mask). (b) Flexible LMA (Ambu AuraFlex disposable laryngeal mask). (c) Second Generation LMA (Ambu AuraGain disposable laryngeal mask). (d) i-gel supraglottic airway. (e) Intubating LMA (LMA Fastrach). Reprinted from [39]. Crown Copyright © 2018 Published by Elsevier Ltd. All rights reserved.

4.3.3 Combined video laryngoscopy and flexible fiberoptic intubation technique

The combination of VL and flexible scope or optical stylet is gaining popularity in complex airway management [40–42]. Video laryngoscopy provides an enlarged view of the glottis and facilitates manipulation of the flexible scope or optical stylet in patients with distorted anatomy or airway tumors. The combined technique allows continuous visualization and reduced trauma to friable tumors or masses.

4.3.4 Surgical airway

Surgical airway is considered when endotracheal intubation fails or when traditional endotracheal intubation is not a feasible option due to the nature and unique requirements of the surgery. Awake tracheostomy under local anesthesia should be strongly considered as a primary plan in patients with significant airway obstruction. It may also be planned as the primary intubation strategy in patients who are expected to have significant airway compromise postoperatively possibly due to extensive reconstructive surgery. An alternative is awake cricothyroidotomy (CTM) which can be safely performed for any patients with difficult airways [43]. In case of emergency airway management, surgical cricothyroidotomy is strongly preferred over the percutaneous cricothyroidotomy as the chance of failure of emergency transcutaneous CTM is nearly 60% in H&N patients according to NAP4 report.

4.3.5 Choice of endotracheal tube

The type and size of tubes depending on the type of surgeries, location, invasiveness of the surgery, and the patient's factors (**Figure 5**). The size and type of ETT should be determined with the surgeon. Endotracheal tubes must be appropriately sized and adequately secured to prevent accidental extubation or displacement during surgery.

- A reinforced, flexible ETT is an excellent choice for shared airway procedures. They are commonly utilized for intraoral surgery.

- Nasal endotracheal intubation (e.g. Nasal RAE tube) is commonly preferred for procedures such as transoral robotic surgery, orthognathic and maxillomandibular surgery, base of tongue surgery, and some dental procedures as it provides better visualization of the oral cavity.

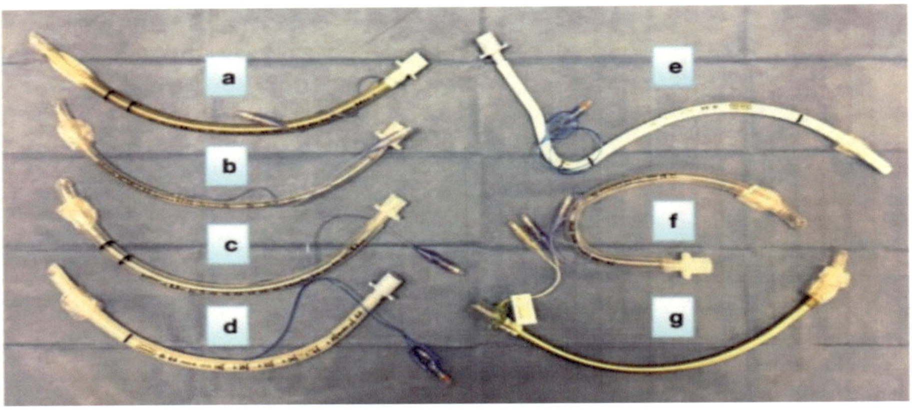

Figure 5.
Tracheal Tubes. (a) Armored flexible (Mallinckrodt Lo-Contour Reinforced TT). (b) Micro laryngeal (Mallinckrodt Microlaryngeal TT Cuffed). (c) Standard (Mallinckrodt Hi-Contour Cuffed TT). (d) Standard Profile Cuff (Portex Profile Soft Seal Cuff). (e) Preformed Polar North Facing Nasal (Portex Ivory PVC, North Facing, Nasal, Profile Soft Seal Cuff, Polar Preformed). (f) Preformed RAE South Facing Oral (Mallinckrodt Oral RAE TT Cuffed). (g) Laser (Mallinckrodt Laser TT Dual Cuffed). Reprinted from [39]. Crown Copyright © 2018 Published by Elsevier Ltd. All rights reserved.

- A small-sized micro laryngeal tube (5-mm internal diameter tube but are longer than standard tube) is commonly used for micro laryngeal surgery to facilitate surgical access.

- A specialized laser-resistant endotracheal tube is used for airway laser surgery.

- Nerve integrity monitor endotracheal tube may be used for specific H&N procedures closely approximating the laryngeal nerves.

4.4 Oxygenation and ventilation strategies

Maintenance of oxygenation and ventilation is the cornerstone of shared airway management in H&N surgery as these patients are at high risk of failed tracheal intubation and a “cannot intubate, cannot ventilate” situation. Traditional methods of increasing the apneic window during induction involve spontaneous facemask ventilation with 100 percent oxygen. Transnasal high-flow rapid insufflation ventilator exchange or THRIVE delivered through a nasal high-flow oxygen delivery system has been shown to increase the apnea time in a patient with difficult airway to an average of 14 minutes (**Figure 6**) [44]. THRIVE provides apneic oxygenation, continuous positive airway pressure to avoid atelectasis, as well as flow-dependent dead space and carbon dioxide flushing, and its role in difficult airway management is presently being studied. Alternatively, a pre-operative transtracheal jet ventilation (TTJV) cannula or an Arndt cricothyroidotomy catheter can be used for tracheal oxygen insufflation [45] to facilitate ventilation. For patients at risk of rapid desaturation or anticipated difficult airway, the provider may use the head-up position, then noninvasive ventilation (NIV) for preoxygenation followed by apneic oxygenation after induction of anesthesia.

Various ventilatory techniques are applied to meet the demands of H&N surgery such as the type of surgery and the access required to the operative site. Following are the ventilator mode techniques used during laryngologic surgery

- **Spontaneous ventilation with local anesthesia or sedation**: this mode of ventilation allows patients to maintain their airways, but few tolerate procedures with such mode of ventilation.

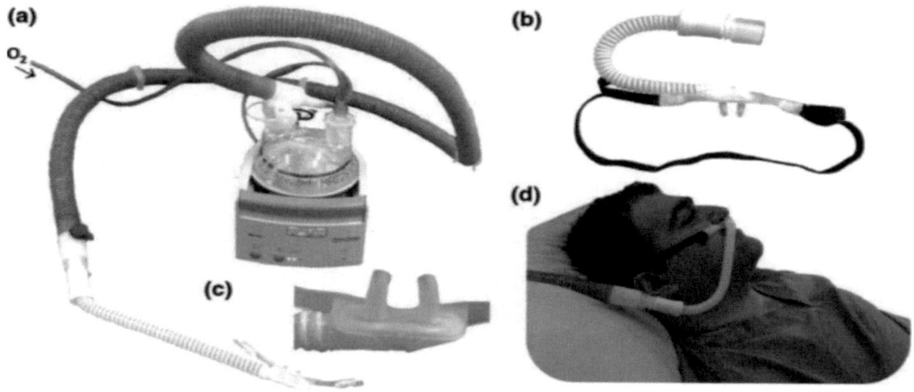

Figure 6.
The OptiFlow high-flow humidified oxygen delivery system. The oxygen humidification unit (a) receives oxygen from a standard oxygen regulator and delivers humidified oxygen to a custom-built transnasal oxygen cannula (b and c) like a standard nasal oxygen cannula (d). Reprinted from [44]. © 2014 The Authors Anaesthesia published by John Wiley & Sons Ltd on behalf of Association of Anaesthetists of Great Britain and Ireland.

Type by technique	Type by location
• Conventional jet ventilation or LFJV (manual via high pressure manual jet)	• Supraglottic (via rigid ENT laryngoscope)
• High Frequency jet ventilation via machine with low tidal volumes and high frequencies	• Subglottic (via special catheter)
	• Trantracheal (via cannula)

Table 5.
Classification of jet ventilation.

- **Spontaneous respiration with general anesthesia**: common in pediatric; oxygenation and ventilation are provided via Stroz bronchoscopy for upper airway endoscopic procedures.

- **Intermittent, Positive-pressure ventilation**: this is usually carried out using a micro laryngoscopy tube (MLT), and allows for the use of standard anesthetic equipment in a normal operating setup. However, it provides a mobile operative field that moves with respiration and sometimes surgical access is reduced or obscured especially in surgery involving the posterior third of the glottis.

- **Intermittent apnea without endotracheal intubation**: this has the advantage of providing an unobstructed surgical view but poor airway protection and inadequate control of anesthesia depth. The patient's airway is intubated in cases of desaturation and but may be extubated prior to surgery resumption.

- **Jet ventilation**: consists of rapid insufflation of gas (oxygen) at high velocity via a narrow nozzle into an open airway. It can be done at either low or high-frequencys. Jet ventilation can be delivered via supraglottic, infraglottic, or transtracheal routes and it provides the optimal surgical view with reduced stimulation (**Table 5**). Paralysis and TIVA are usually required for this technique.

i. **Low-frequency jet ventilation** (LFJV) is delivered using a high-pressure gas source via a narrow cannula attached to a suspension laryngoscope or bronchoscope. Ventilatory frequency is usually around 10–30 cycles per minute. The stream of high-velocity gas entrains air and increases the tidal volume but reduces the oxygen concentration of the inspired gas. It is easy to perform, requiring uncomplicated anesthetic equipment and allows a clear surgical view. Inhalational anesthesia may not be delivered easily, so total intravenous anesthesia is preferred. However, there are certain disadvantages such as mobility of the operative field, difficulty monitoring airway pressure, risk of gas entrainment, and barotrauma

ii. **High-frequency jet ventilation** is more commonly used especially for infraglottic and transtracheal routes. HFJV is usually set at 150 cycles per minute, delivering tidal volumes as small as 1 to 3 ml/kg. HFJV provides a motionless and still surgical field. TIVA is the anesthesia of choice. However, there are possible risks of gastric insufflation, carbon dioxide retention, and barotrauma

4.5 Analgesia

A multimodal approach in the form of acetaminophen, non-steroidal anti-inflammatory drugs, gabapentin, opioids, and local as well as regional anesthesia can be given perioperatively. Post-operative patient-controlled analgesia can be considered with step down to oral opioids as required.

4.6 Postoperative nausea and vomiting (PONV) prophylaxis

Patients who undergo H&N surgery are at high risk of postoperative nausea and vomiting and should be managed aggressively as it can result in increased morbidity. A multimodal approach to prophylaxis is essential, encompassing TIVA with intraoperative dexamethasone (8 mg Intravenous), 5-HT3 antagonist (e.g. ondansetron 4 to 8 mg intravenous), and utilization of multimodal analgesia to minimize opioid requirement.

Classes of antiemetics are

- 5-HT3 receptor antagonists (e.g. ondansetron)
- Nk-1 receptor antagonists (e.g. aprepitant)
- Corticosteroids (e.g. dexamethasone)
- Butyrophenones (e.g. haloperidol)
- Antihistamines (e.g. meclizine)
- Anticholinergics (e.g. scopolamine)
- Phenothiazines (e.g., metoclopramide)

4.7 Emergence and extubation

The goals of safe emergence from anesthesia include smooth, rapid emergence and extubation, avoidance of straining, bucking, and coughing, and a complete, pain-free awakening. Extubation plan should be formulated thoroughly with the surgeons in the preoperative period. One may consider the extubation guidelines as outlined by the Difficult Airway Society of the United Kingdom or American Society of Anesthesiologists Practice Guidelines for the management of the difficult airway [46, 47]. In cases of anticipated post-operative airway complications, extubation may be delayed and patient should be transported to the intensive care unit. Extubation considerations should include the following options:

- Fully awaken the patient and extubate immediately postoperatively
- If anticipating airway compromise, admit to the intensive care unit for a delayed tracheal extubation
- Conduct tracheostomy.

5. Postoperative management

Enhanced recovery after surgery protocol should be applied to facilitate fast-track discharge as most of the H&N surgeries are done on an ambulatory basis [19]. Those patients who require post-operative airway management should be cared for in intensive care unit. Varadarajan and colleagues [48] proposed that any of the following could be indications for postoperative ICU admission:

- Patients requiring post-op assisted ventilation
- Patients requiring diagnostic or therapeutic bronchoscopy
- Patients requiring invasive hemodynamic or cardiac monitoring such as in the setting of hemodynamic instability
- Patients with multiorgan failure requiring critical care management.

6. Special considerations

6.1 Anesthesia considerations for transoral robotic surgery (TORS)

Transoral robotic surgery is a minimally invasive surgical technique most widely used for radical tonsillectomy, oropharyngeal cancer resection, localization of occult primary head and neck tumors, supraglottic partial laryngectomy, and treatment of snoring and obstructive sleep apnea [49]. TORS allows exceptional surgical treatment of head and neck pathology while minimizing morbidity and improving functional outcomes as compared with open surgical approaches. Anesthetic challenges include shared airway with a robot and limited access to the patient intraoperatively. Airway management includes nasal RAE or wire-reinforced endotracheal intubation and the use of TIVA with a combination of TCI propofol and remifentanil as the choice of anesthetic. Possible complications include pressure point injury and deep vein thrombosis due to prolonged surgery, risk of airway fire, aspiration, and post-operative bleeding. As TORS expands, local guidelines must be produced that support high standards of perioperative care [49, 50].

6.2 Anesthesia considerations for laser surgery

Laser surgery is employed to treat laryngeal pathoses such as papilloma, laryngomalacia, vocal cord cysts, vocal cord polyps and granulomas, and post-operative scar tissues. Laser micro laryngoscopy enables precise management of a wide range of upper airway conditions. The type of airway management required for laser surgery is determined by whether access is needed to the hypopharynx, supraglottis, larynx, or subglottis. Ventilatory techniques that may be used include continuous endotracheal intubation with specialized laser tubes, spontaneous ventilation with insufflation techniques, intermittent apneic technique, or jet ventilation (supraglottic or subglottic) and with TIVA. TIVA using propofol and remifentanil titrated to maintain spontaneous ventilation is an alternative technique. Laser-resistant endotracheal tubes are used as airway fire poses a major risk. For a fire to occur, the triad of fuel (e.g., ETT, drapes, sponges), oxygen, and ignition source is needed. The American Society of Anesthesiologists (ASA) published an operating room fire algorithm that guides managing airway fires [51]:

- Declare a fire and alert the team
- Halt the procedure and the laser beam
- Irrigate the surgical field with saline
- Immediately cease airway gases/ventilation and remove ETT
- Remove sponge and other flammable materials from the airway
- Resume bag-mask ventilation and prepare for reintubation once the airway fire is extinguished
- Examine the airway for evidence of debris, thermal injury, or foreign bodies and consider bronchoscopy

6.3 Anesthesia considerations for endoscopic sinus surgery

Functional endoscopic sinus surgery is an effective, low-risk procedure for chronic rhinosinusitis, nasal polyposis, epistaxis control, tumor excision, foreign body removal, treatment of sinus mucoceles, and more. Anesthetic considerations include local versus general anesthesia, supraglottic airway devices versus endotracheal intubation, inhaled anesthesia versus TIVA, and the preferences of the surgical team while taking the patient's comorbidities into account. The main goals are to provide a bloodless surgical field, patient immobility, stable hemodynamic conditions, and smooth emergence. Different techniques are utilized to induce "controlled hypotension" which reduces bleeding and improves the surgical visual field. However, this procedure has potential major complications which include orbital hematoma resulting in blindness or reduced vision, cerebrospinal fluid leaks, renal or arterial injury, severe hemorrhage, and death.

6.4 Anesthesia consideration for major oral and maxillofacial cancer surgery

Because oral cancers are associated with smoking and alcohol excess, cardiopulmonary compromise and malnutrition are more common comorbidities. Moreover, airway difficulty can arise due to distortion of the airway by the tumor or as a consequence of radiotherapy. Surgery is typically performed using general anesthesia with tracheal intubation (preferably nasal ETT) and invasive hemodynamic monitors depending on the extent of the surgery and the patient's comorbidities. Hypotensive anesthesia is encouraged to reduce blood loss. Long-acting paralytics should be avoided when electromyography is employed, TIVA is often a preferred anesthetic choice. The application of ERAS to major head and neck cancer surgery has led to other guidelines for perioperative management.

6.5 Anesthesia consideration for free flap transfer

Tissue transfer in the form of a pedicled or microvascular free flap is commonly employed to reconstruct defects following H&N cancer resection [52]. The graft may consist of soft tissues, bone, or both. Anesthetic management aims to maintain a full, hyperdynamic circulation with increased cardiac output, liberal fluid resuscitation, peripheral vasodilation, and normothermia to maximize flap perfusion. Hematocrit should be maintained at 30–35% to improve oxygen transfer and red cell velocity within the microcirculation. Vasoconstrictors are usually discouraged as they can contribute to graft ischemia. Intraoperative and postoperative flap monitoring is achieved clinically (by bedside examination of the flap color, temperature, turgor, edema, and capillary refill), and by using technical means such as Doppler ultrasound or near-infrared spectroscopy.

6.6 Anesthesia consideration for craniofacial surgery

Craniofacial surgery addresses congenital or acquired deformities through cleft lip and palate repair, temporomandibular joint surgery, and orthognathic procedures. Obstructive sleep apnea and congenital airway deformormities is common in these patients. In general, nasal intubation is frequently preferred in orthognathic surgery. Submental intubation may be required if the nasal route is difficult or if the surgeon requires access to the upper portion of the face. In submental intubation, an incision is first made through the submental skin into the floor of the mouth. After routine oral intubation, the proximal end of the endotracheal tube is passed through the floor of the mouth out to the submental skin. The process is reversed at the end of the surgery and the patient is extubated orally. Bleeding is a potential risk that can be controlled by positioning the patient head up, ensuring free venous drainage, utilizing local anesthesia containing adrenaline, and utilizing controlled hypotension. Antibiotic prophylaxis, multi-modal analgesia, PONV prophylaxis, and steroids to reduce swelling are also important components of perioperative management.

7. Virtual endoscopy and 3-D reconstruction for airway evaluation in H&N pathology

Preemptive imaging of the airway is a valuable aide to traditional clinical airway evaluation for strategizing airway management. The NAP4 highlighted that 40% of the patients with head and neck pathology developed airway related complications. These failures were attributed to shortcomings in airway evaluation, planning, and adaptations of airway and anesthetic techniques according to the patient's pathology. Virtual endoscopy (VE) has been utilized by radiologists for many years to assess, identify, and stage the various lesions. VE utilizes multidimensional CT images to construct 3D endoscopic images at various sites from the nasopharynx to a tracheobronchial tree [53]. VE enables computer-generated 3-dimensional portrayal of the airway cavity (**Figures 7–9**). Virtual endoscopy is a valuable and safe tool as it provides a complete, non-invasive, and anatomically accurate portrayal of the patient's airway, starting from nasopharynx or oro-pharynx to the tracheobronchial tree. The virtual airway can be reconstructed from the patient's pre-existing diagnostic CT images using the OsiriX software [54–56]. VE can contribute significantly to preemptive strategies against the NAP4 highlighted shortcomings and help improve overall patient outcome.

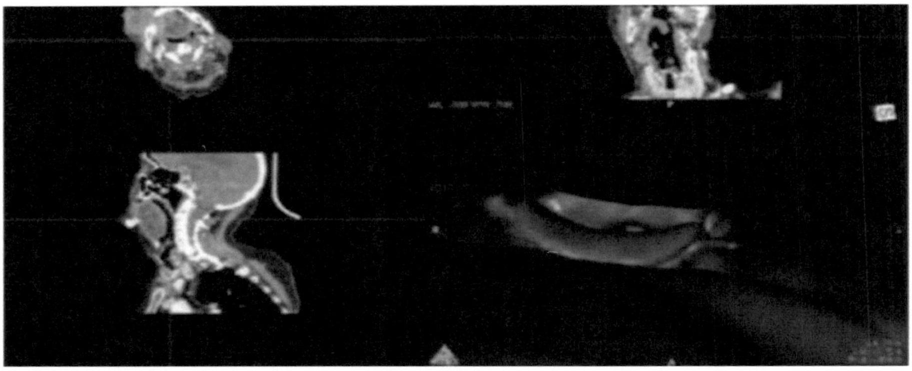

Figure 7.
Supraglottic virtual endoscopy reconstruction showing the epiglottis [54]. Reprinted with permission from Dr. Imran Ahmad FRCA, Consultant Anaesthetist, Clinical Lead for Airway Management, Service Clinical Lead for Anaesthesia & Theatres, Guy's Hospital, Guy's & St Thomas' NHS Foundation Trust, London, UK & Honorary Senior Lecturer, King's College London, UK.

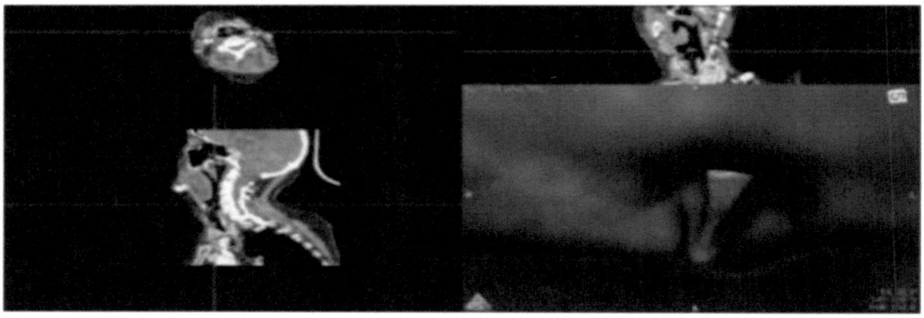

Figure 8.
Virtual endoscopy reconstruction showing the glottic opening [54]. Reprinted with permission from Dr. Imran Ahmad FRCA, Consultant Anaesthetist, Clinical Lead for Airway.

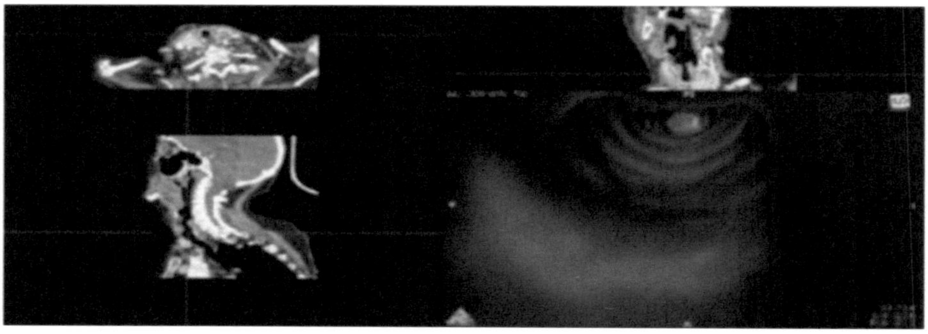

Figure 9.
Subglottic virtual endoscopy reconstruction showing the trachea [54]. Reprinted with permission from Dr. Imran Ahmad FRCA, Consultant Anaesthetist, Clinical Lead for Airway Management, Service Clinical Lead for Anaesthesia & Theatres, Guy's Hospital, Guy's & St Thomas' NHS Foundation Trust, London, UK & Honorary Senior Lecturer, King's College London, UK.

8. The COVID-19 pandemic and head and neck surgery

The novel coronavirus disease 2019 (COVID-19) has become a pandemic exposing many unprecedented challenges to health care systems. In head and neck procedures, health care staff are at a higher risk of contracting the virus as most examinations and procedures within the respiratory tract. Understanding how to mitigate the risks is critical. The British Otolaryngology Society and the American Society of Gastrointestinal Endoscopy recommended mandatory personal protective equipment (PPE) use, procedures performed in negative-pressure rooms, and thorough decontamination of endoscopes, equipment, and rooms. All non-urgent surgery should be deferred to prevent consumption of emergency equipment and avoid outpatients spread. Airway management strategies should include designating experienced providers, closing circuits, intubating in negative pressure rooms, applying rapid sequence induction techniques, and minimizing bag-mask ventilation. All standard airway equipments should be available including bag-masks with High-Efficiency Particular Air (HEPA) filters, video laryngoscopes with disposable blades, ventilators, and tubes with inline adapter, HEPA filter, and clamp for ETT for application during tube disconnection to avoid aerosolization [57]. On the other hand, awake intubation should be avoided as coughing and bucking may promote aerosolization. THRIVE, jet ventilation, or open-circuit positive pressure ventilation are discouraged. Laser surgery or endonasal and otologic drilling should be avoided as viral particles can spread through plumes [58].

9. Conclusion

Head and neck surgery involves a wide range of procedures from the simple to the complex. Thus, it poses greater challenges to the anesthesiologist; he/she must optimize the patient's comorbidities preoperatively, share the airway, implement different anesthesia and airway techniques specific to each surgery, and manage postoperative airway complications. Head and neck surgery patients often present with difficult airways due to the pathologies which impede the airway anatomy. Therefore, preoperative planning necessitates thorough history and physical examination with particular attention to the airway evaluation. High-risk patients should be identified preoperatively and medically optimized before surgery. A multidisciplinary approach and expertise in H&N anesthesia and advanced airway management should be encouraged as it decreases airway complications and improves surgical outcomes. The preoperative endoscopic airway examination is a useful aide in providing a real-time image of the upper airway and allows adequate preparation. General anesthesia with total intravenous anesthesia (TIVA) is the anesthesia of choice as it offers quick titration of anesthesia, allows immobility, prevents postoperative nausea and vomiting, reduces blood loss by inducing controlled hypotension, and facilitates smooth and rapid emergence. Airway management planning also requires close communication and cooperation with the surgical team. Endotracheal intubation is a general considered in H&N surgery because it offers optimal airway control with adequate oxygenation, ventilation, and protection against aspiration. Video laryngoscopy is recommended in H&N surgery. Different ventilator techniques including jet ventilation should be considered in H&N surgery. Furthermore, multimodal analgesia, PONV prophylaxis, use of steroids to reduce airway edema, and antibiotic prophylaxis are essential components of intraoperative management. Enhanced recovery after surgery (ERAS) guidelines in H&N surgery should be applied. The decision to admit a patient in the critical care unit postoperatively is based on the patient's comorbidities, intraoperative events, complexities of the surgery, and requirements for airway support. Recent advances in airway management techniques (such as virtual endoscopy) and surgical techniques have been shown to improve the outcome.

Conflict of interest

The authors declare no conflict of interest.

Author details

Muhammad Jaffar Khan*, Tarek Tageldin, Muhammad Waqas Farooqi, Odai Qasim Khamash, Umair Shahid, Mohamed El-Fatih Abdul-Rahman, Mohamed Elarref and Jazib Hassan
Department of Anesthesia, Perioperative Medicine and Critical Care, Hamad Medical Corporation, Doha, Qatar

*Address all correspondence to: jafar06khan@gmail.com

References

[1] Cook TM, Woodall N, Harper J, Benger J. Major complications of airway management in the UK: Results of the Fourth National Audit Project of the Royal College of Anaesthetists and the Difficult Airway Society. Part 2: Intensive care and emergency departments. Br J Anaesth. 2011;

[2] Patel A, Pearce A P, P. Chapter 18 Head and neck pathology. In: Fourth National Audit Project of the Royal College of Anaesthetists and Difficult Airway Society. 2011. p. 143-154.

[3] Rosenstock C V., Nørskov AK, Wetterslev J, Lundstrøm LH. Emergency surgical airway management in Denmark: A cohort study of 452 461 patients registered in the Danish Anaesthesia Database. Br J Anaesth [Internet]. 2016 Sep 1 [cited 2020 Sep 24];117:i75-82. Available from: http://bjanaesthesia.org/article/S0007091217337716/fulltext

[4] Arné J, Descoins P, Fusciardi J, Ferrier B, Boudigues D, Ariès J. Preoperative assessment for difficult intubation in general and ENT surgery: predictive value of a clinical multivariate risk index †. Vol. 80, British Journal of Anaesthesia. 1998.

[5] Iseli TA, Iseli CE, Golden JB, Jones VL, Boudreaux AM, Boyce JR, et al. Outcomes of intubation in difficult airways due to head and neck pathology. Ear, Nose Throat J [Internet]. 2012 Mar 10 [cited 2020 Sep 24];91(3):E1-5. Available from: http://journals.sagepub.com/doi/10.1177/014556131209100313

[6] Heinrich S, Birkholz T, Irouschek A, Ackermann A, Schmidt J. Incidences and predictors of difficult laryngoscopy in adult patients undergoing general anesthesia: A single-center analysis of 102,305 cases. J Anesth [Internet]. 2013 Dec 9 [cited 2020 Sep 24];27(6):815-21. Available from: https://link.springer.com/article/10.1007/s00540-013-1650-4

[7] Crosby ET, Cooper RM, Douglas MJ, Doyle DJ, Hung OR, Labrecquc P, et al. The unanticipated difficult airway with recommendations for management. Can J Anaesth [Internet]. 1998 [cited 2020 Sep 24];45(8):757-76. Available from: https://link.springer.com/article/10.1007/BF03012147

[8] Connelly NR, Ghandour K, Robbins L, Dunn S, Gibson C. Management of unexpected difficult airway at a teaching institution over a 7-year period. J Clin Anesth. 2006 May 1;18(3):198-204.

[9] O'Dell K. Predictors of Difficult Intubation and the Otolaryngology Perioperative Consult [Internet]. Vol. 33, Anesthesiology Clinics. W.B. Saunders; 2015 [cited 2020 Sep 24]. p. 279-90. Available from: http://www.anesthesiology.theclinics.com/article/S1932227515000142/fulltext

[10] Cavallone LF, Vannucci A. Extubation of the Difficult Airway and Extubation Failure. Anesth Analg [Internet]. 2013 Feb [cited 2020 Sep 24];116(2):368-83. Available from: http://journals.lww.com/00000539-201302000-00018

[11] Lundstrøm LH, Møller AM, Rosenstock C, Astrup G, Gätke MR, Wetterslev J. A documented previous difficult tracheal intubation as a prognostic test for a subsequent difficult tracheal intubation in adults. Anaesthesia [Internet]. 2009 Oct 1 [cited 2020 Sep 24];64(10):1081-8. Available from: http://doi.wiley.com/10.1111/j.1365-2044.2009.06057.x

[12] Schaeuble JC, Caldwell JE. Effective Communication of Difficult Airway Management to Subsequent Anesthesia Providers.

Anesth Analg [Internet]. 2009 Aug [cited 2020 Sep 24];109(2):684-6. Available from: http://journals.lww.com/00000539-200908000-00063

[13] Brucker JL, Gentry LR. Imaging of Head and Neck Emergencies [Internet]. Vol. 53, Radiologic Clinics of North America. W.B. Saunders; 2015 [cited 2020 Sep 24]. p. 215-52. Available from: http://www.radiologic.theclinics.com/article/S0033838914001468/fulltext

[14] Kheterpal S, Martin L, Shanks AM, Tremper KK. Prediction and outcomes of impossible mask ventilation: A review of 50,000 anesthetics. Anesthesiology [Internet]. 2009 Apr 1 [cited 2020 Sep 1];110(4):891-7. Available from: www.anesthesiology.org.

[15] Apfelbaum JL, Hagberg CA, Caplan RA, Connis RT, Nickinovich DG, Benumof JL, et al. Practice guidelines for management of the difficult airway: An updated report by the American Society of Anesthesiologists Task Force on Management of the Difficult Airway [Internet]. Vol. 118, Anesthesiology. American Society of Anesthesiologists; 2013 [cited 2020 Sep 24]. p. 251-70. Available from: http://links.lww.com/ALN/A902.

[16] Lundstrøm LH, Vester-Andersen M, Møller AM, Charuluxananan S, L'Hermite J, Wetterslev J. Poor prognostic value of the modified Mallampati score: A meta-analysis involving 177 088 patients [Internet]. Vol. 107, British Journal of Anaesthesia. Oxford University Press; 2011 [cited 2020 Sep 24]. p. 659-67. Available from: http://bjanaesthesia.org/article/S0007091217325990/fulltext

[17] Kheterpal S, Healy D, Aziz MF, Shanks AM, Freundlich RE, Linton F, et al. Incidence, predictors, and outcome of difficult mask ventilation combined with difficult laryngoscopy: a report from the multicenter perioperative outcomes group. Anesthesiology [Internet]. 2013 Dec 1 [cited 2020 Sep 24];119(6):1360-9. Available from: http://pubs.asahq.org/anesthesiology/article-pdf/119/6/1360/263731/20131200_0-00022.pdf

[18] Daodu O, Panda N, Lopushinsky S, Varghese TK, Brindle M. COVID-19 – Considerations and Implications for Surgical Learners. Ann Surg [Internet]. 2020 Jul 1 [cited 2020 Aug 24];272(1):e22-3. Available from: https://journals.lww.com/10.1097/SLA.0000000000003927

[19] Coyle MJ, Main B, Hughes C, Craven R, Alexander R, Porter G, et al. Enhanced recovery after surgery (ERAS) for head and neck oncology patients. Clin Otolaryngol [Internet]. 2016 Apr 1 [cited 2020 Sep 24];41(2):118-26. Available from: http://doi.wiley.com/10.1111/coa.12482

[20] ASA: American Society of Anesthesiologist. Standards for Basic Anesthetic Monitoring | American Society of Anesthesiologists (ASA) [Internet]. 2015 [cited 2020 Aug 24]. Available from: https://www.asahq.org/standards-and-guidelines/standards-for-basic-anesthetic-monitoring

[21] Dort JC, Farwell DG, Findlay M, Huber GF, Kerr P, Shea-Budgell MA, et al. Optimal perioperative care in major head and neck cancer surgery with free flap reconstruction: A consensus review and recommendations from the enhanced recovery after surgery society [Internet]. Vol. 143, JAMA Otolaryngology - Head and Neck Surgery. American Medical Association; 2017 [cited 2020 Sep 24]. p. 292-303. Available from: https://jamanetwork.com/journals/jamaotolaryngology/fullarticle/2565537

[22] Eberhart LHJ, Eberspaecher M, Wulf H, Geldner G. Fast-track eligibility, costs and quality of recovery after intravenous anaesthesia with propofol-remifentanil versus balanced

anaesthesia with isoflurane-alfentanil. Eur J Anaesthesiol [Internet]. 2004 Feb [cited 2020 Sep 24];21(2):107-14. Available from: /core/journals/european-journal-of-anaesthesiology/article/fasttrack-eligibility-costs-and-quality-of-recovery-after-intravenous-anaesthesia-with-propofolremifentanil-versus-balanced-anaesthesia-with-isofluranealfentanil/2463B3205297D3F2B8DEF68670E1B135

[23] Brunner JP, Levy JM, Ada ML, Tipirneni KE, Barham HP, Oakley GM, et al. Total intravenous anesthesia improves intraoperative visualization during surgery for high-grade chronic rhinosinusitis: a double-blind randomized controlled trial. Int Forum Allergy Rhinol [Internet]. 2018 Oct 1 [cited 2020 Sep 5]; 8(10):1114-22. Available from: http://doi.wiley.com/10.1002/alr.22173

[24] Mort TC. Emergency Tracheal Intubation: Complications Associated with Repeated Laryngoscopic Attempts. Anesth Analg [Internet]. 2004 Aug [cited 2020 Sep 1];99(2):607-13. Available from: http://journals.lww.com/00000539-200408000-00056

[25] Kelly FE, Cook TM. Seeing is believing: Getting the best out of videolaryngoscopy [Internet]. Vol. 117, British Journal of Anaesthesia. Oxford University Press; 2016 [cited 2020 Sep 1]. p. i9-13. Available from: https://academic.oup.com/bja/article/117/suppl_1/i9/1744017

[26] Griesdale DEG, Liu D, McKinney J, Choi PT. Glidescope ® video-laryngoscopy versus direct laryngoscopy for endotracheal intubation: A systematic review and meta-analysis. Can J Anesth [Internet]. 2012 Jan 1 [cited 2020 Sep 1];59(1):41-52. Available from: https://link.springer.com/article/10.1007/s12630-011-9620-5

[27] Aziz MF, Healy D, Kheterpal S, Fu RF, Dillman D, Brambrink AM. Routine clinical practice effectiveness of the glidescope in difficult airway management: An analysis of 2,004 glidescope intubations, complications, and failures from two institutions. Anesthesiology [Internet]. 2011 Jan 1 [cited 2020 Sep 1];114(1):34-41. Available from: http://pubs.asahq.org/anesthesiology/article-pdf/114/1/34/252877/0000542-201101000-00017.pdf

[28] Mason RA, Fielder CP. The obstructed airway in head and neck surgery. Anaesthesia [Internet]. 1999 Jul 1 [cited 2020 Sep 1];54(7):625-8. Available from: http://doi.wiley.com/10.1046/j.1365-2044.1999.01036.x

[29] Iseli TA, Iseli CE, Golden JB, Jones VL, Boudreaux AM, Boyce JR, et al. Outcomes of intubation in difficult airways due to head and neck pathology. Ear, Nose Throat J [Internet]. 2012 Mar 10 [cited 2020 Sep 1];91(3):E1-5. Available from: http://journals.sagepub.com/doi/10.1177/014556131209100313

[30] MacMillan, M.H. and Davidson, M. (2020) 'Anaesthesia for endoscopic surgery', Anaesthesia and Intensive Care Medicine. Elsevier Ltd, pp. 205-208. doi: 10.1016/j.mpaic.2020.01.006. 2020

[31] Apfelbaum JL, Hagberg CA, Caplan RA, Connis RT, Nickinovich DG, Benumof JL, et al. Practice guidelines for management of the difficult airway: An updated report by the American Society of Anesthesiologists Task Force on Management of the Difficult Airway [Internet]. Vol. 118, Anesthesiology. American Society of Anesthesiologists; 2013 [cited 2020 Sep 1]. p. 251-70. Available from: http://links.lww.com/ALN/A902.

[32] Benjamin B, Lindholm CE. Systematic direct laryngoscopy: The Lindholm laryngoscopes. Ann Otol Rhinol Laryngol [Internet]. 2003 Sep 29 [cited 2020 Sep 1];112(9 I):787-97. Available from: http://journals.sagepub.com/doi/10.1177/000348940311200908

[33] Davies R, Balachandran S. Anterior commissure laryngoscope. Anaesthesia [Internet]. 2003 Jul 1 [cited 2020 Sep 1];58(7):721-2. Available from: http://doi.wiley.com/10.1046/j.1365-2044.2003.327713.x

[34] Hillel AT, Pandian V, Mark LJ, Clark J, Miller CR, Haut ER, et al. A novel role for otolaryngologists in the multidisciplinary difficult airway response team. Laryngoscope [Internet]. 2015 Mar 1 [cited 2020 Sep 1];125(3):640-4. Available from: http://doi.wiley.com/10.1002/lary.24949

[35] Nekhendzy V, Simmonds PK. Rigid Bronchoscope-Assisted Endotracheal Intubation: Yet Another Use of the Gum Elastic Bougie. Anesth Analg [Internet]. 2004 Feb [cited 2020 Sep 1];98(2):545-7. Available from: http://journals.lww.com/00000539-200402000-00051

[36] Nowakowski M, Williams S, Gallant J, Ruel M, Robitaille A. Predictors of Difficult Intubation with the Bonfils Rigid Fiberscope. Anesth Analg [Internet]. 2016 Jun 1 [cited 2020 Sep 1];122(6):1901-6. Available from: http://journals.lww.com/00000539-201606000-00028

[37] Corbanese U, Morossi M. The Bonfils intubation fibrescope: clinical evaluation and consideration of the learning curve. Eur J Anaesthesiol [Internet]. 2009 Jul [cited 2020 Sep 1];26(7):622-4. Available from: http://journals.lww.com/00003643-200907000-00018

[38] Aziz M, Metz S. Clinical evaluation of the Levitan Optical Stylet*. Anaesthesia [Internet]. 2011 Jul 1 [cited 2020 Sep 1];66(7):579-81. Available from: http://doi.wiley.com/10.1111/j.1365-2044.2011.06708.x

[39] Laurie, A., & Macdonald, J. (2018). Equipment for airway management. Anaesthesia & Intensive Care Medicine, 19(8), 389-396

[40] Sharma D, Kim LJ, Ghodke B. Successful airway management with combined use of glidescope® videolaryngoscope and fiberoptic bronchoscope in a patient with cowden syndrome. Anesthesiology [Internet]. 2010 Jul 1 [cited 2020 Sep 1];113(1):253-5. Available from: http://pubs.asahq.org/anesthesiology/article-pdf/113/1/253/250530/0000542-201007000-00035.pdf

[41] Gu J, Xu K, Ning J, Yi B, Lu K. GlideScope-assisted fiberoptic bronchoscope intubation in a patient with severe rheumatoid arthritis. Acta Anaesthesiol Taiwanica. 2014 Jun 1;52(2):85-7.

[42] Vieira FO, Rhodes CB, Smith A, Case CRNA S. Videolaryngoscope Assisted Fiberoptic Bronchoscopy for Difficult Intubation in Upper Airway Cancer. Res Artic. 2018;14(3).

[43] Boyce JR, Peters GE, Carroll WR, Magnuson JS, McCrory A, Boudreaux AM. Preemptive vessel dilator cricothyrotomy aids in the management of upper airway obstruction [Internet]. Vol. 52, Canadian Journal of Anesthesia. Canadian Anaesthetists' Society; 2005 [cited 2020 Sep 1]. p. 765-9. Available from: https://link.springer.com/article/10.1007/BF03016567

[44] Patel A, Nouraei SAR. Transnasal Humidified Rapid-Insufflation Ventilatory Exchange (THRIVE): a physiological method of increasing apnoea time in patients with difficult airways. Anaesthesia [Internet]. 2015 Mar 1 [cited 2020 Sep 5];70(3):323-9. Available from: http://doi.wiley.com/10.1111/anae.12923

[45] Roberts J, Barrass L, Hunningher A. Arndt airway can contribute to the elective management of difficult airway cases [Internet]. Vol. 107, British Journal of Anaesthesia. Oxford University Press; 2011 [cited 2020 Sep 5]. p. 470. Available from: http://bjanaesthesia.org/article/S000709121733088X/fulltext

[46] Ogilvie L. Difficult Airway Society guidelines for the management of tracheal extubation. Anaesthesia [Internet]. 2012 Nov 1 [cited 2020 Sep 5];67(11):1277-8. Available from: http://doi.wiley.com/10.1111/anae.12011

[47] Apfelbaum JL, Hagberg CA, Caplan RA, Connis RT, Nickinovich DG, Benumof JL, et al. Practice guidelines for management of the difficult airway: An updated report by the American Society of Anesthesiologists Task Force on Management of the Difficult Airway [Internet]. Vol. 118, Anesthesiology. American Society of Anesthesiologists; 2013 [cited 2020 Sep 5]. p. 251-70. Available from: http://links.lww.com/ALN/A902.

[48] Varadarajan V V., Arshad H, Dziegielewski PT. Head and neck free flap reconstruction: What is the appropriate post-operative level of care? Oral Oncol. 2017 Dec 1;75:61-6.

[49] Dinsmore JE. Anaesthetic Considerations for Transoral Robotic Surgery (TORS) [Internet]. 2018 [cited 2020 Sep 5]. Available from: www.wfsahq.org/resources/anaesthesia-tutorial-of-the-week

[50] Chi JJ, Mandel JE, Weinstein GS, O'Malley BW. Anesthetic Considerations for Transoral Robotic Surgery [Internet]. Vol. 28, Anesthesiology Clinics. Elsevier; 2010 [cited 2020 Sep 5]. p. 411-22. Available from: http://www.anesthesiology.theclinics.com/article/S193222751000056X/fulltext

[51] Apfelbaum JL, Caplan RA, Connis RT, Ehrenwerth J, Nickinovich DG, Pritchard D, et al. Practice advisory for the prevention and management of operating room fires: An updated report by the American Society of Anesthesiologists Task Force on Operating room fires. Anesthesiology [Internet]. 2013 Feb 1 [cited 2020 Sep 5];118(2):271-90. Available from: http://pubs.asahq.org/anesthesiology/article-pdf/118/2/271/261099/20130200_0-00013.pdf

[52] Pereira CMB, Figueiredo MEL, Carvalho R, Catre D, Assunção JP. Anesthesia and Surgical Microvascular Flaps. Vol. 62, Revista Brasileira de Anestesiologia. Elsevier; 2012. p. 563-79.

[53] De Wever W, Vandecaveye V, Lanciotti S, Verschakelen JA. Multidetector CT-generated virtual bronchoscopy: An illustrated review of the potential clinical indications [Internet]. Vol. 23, European Respiratory Journal. European Respiratory Society; 2004 [cited 2020 Sep 22]. p. 776-82. Available from: https://erj.ersjournals.com/content/23/5/776

[54] Ahmad I, Keane O, Muldoon S. Enhancing airway assessment of patients with head and neck pathology using virtual endoscopy. Indian J Anaesth [Internet]. 2017 Oct 1 [cited 2020 Sep 22];61(10):782. Available from: http://www.ijaweb.org/text.asp?2017/61/10/782/216676

[55] Fried MP, Moharir VM, Lorensen WE, Shinmoto H, Hsu L, Alyassin AM, et al. Virtual laryngoscopy. Ann Otol Rhinol Laryngol [Internet]. 1999 Mar 28 [cited 2020 Sep 22];108(3):221-6. Available from: http://journals.sagepub.com/doi/10.1177/000348949910800301

[56] Ahmad I, Millhoff B, John M, Andi K, Oakley R. Virtual endoscopy - A new assessment tool in difficult airway management. J Clin Anesth. 2015 Sep 1;27(6):508-13.

[57] Wax RS, Christian MD. Practical recommendations for critical care and anesthesiology teams caring for novel coronavirus (2019-nCoV) patients [Internet]. Vol. 67, Canadian Journal of Anesthesia. Springer;

2020 [cited 2020 Sep 21]. p. 568-76. Available from: https://doi.org/10.1007/s12630-020-01591-x

[58] Couloigner V, Schmerber S, Nicollas R, Coste A, Barry B, Makeieff M, et al. COVID-19 and ENT Surgery. Eur Ann Otorhinolaryngol Head Neck Dis. 2020 May 1;137(3):161-6.

Chapter 6

Surgical Treatment of Velopharyngeal Insufficiency

Nguyen Pham and Isabella Rodoni

Abstract

Velopharyngeal insufficiency (VPI) is a condition where the soft palate and posterior oropharynx fail to close adequately, leading to complications such as abnormal speech, nasal regurgitation and nasal emission. Although there exist many approaches to treating VPI depending on the shape and severity of the insufficiency, this chapter describes the three most frequently used and well-researched techniques: the Furlow Palatoplasty (double-opposing Z-palatoplasty), the creation and placement of a pharyngeal flap, and a sphincter pharyngoplasty. This chapter contains an introduction to VPI causes and treatment, a description of patient assessment methods, step-by-step instructions for the different operative procedures, and the recovery process.

Keywords: cleft surgery, craniofacial, cleft palate, velopharyngeal, pharyngeal flap, furlow palatoplasty, VPI

1. Introduction

The velopharyngeal sphincter separates the nasopharynx from the oropharynx and is located where the soft palate meets the posterior oropharyngeal wall. When functioning properly, the velopharyngeal sphincter closes and opens to allow appropriate air flow for normal speech, eating, and breathing. The sphincter closes to stop airflow up to the nasal cavity for consonant pronunciation and to prevent nasal regurgitation. It opens to produce certain nasal vocalizations and for normal breathing. Velopharyngeal Insufficiency (VPI) occurs when the sphincter cannot close completely and can cause hypernasality, nasal emissions, nasal regurgitation of food and liquid and communication difficulties.

VPI is usually caused by a complete or submucous cleft palate. An estimated 5–30% of patients continue to have VPI post-cleft palate repair [1]. Temporary VPI can also occur following adenoidectomy. Children with velocardiofacial syndrome (DiGeorge Syndrome) can suffer from VPI without a cleft palate. Lastly, traumatic brain injury or neurological disorders can cause VPI due to muscle weakness or difficulty coordinating palatal muscles. Depending on the anatomy of the velopharyngeal gap, there are different surgical approaches to treatment. Possibilities for surgery include Furlow Double Opposing Z-Palatoplasty, sphincter pharyngoplasty, posterior pharyngeal wall injection, or pharyngeal flap pharyngoplasty. These approaches vary based on availability of flap tissue-source, individual closure pattern, and severity of VPI. A surgeon needs to be able to distinguish between each technique's risks and benefits before operating; VPI is expressed differently in every patient, therefore surgical approaches will benefit each patient differently. Correcting VPI can help a patient to gain the ability to effectively communicate, as well as their confidence in doing so by minimizing emissions and improving intelligibility [2, 3].

2. Speech and sphincter assessment

Children with cleft palate are at high risk of developing VPI and should be routinely assessed by a speech pathologist experienced in the management of VPI. Most cases of VPI in the cleft population resolve with speech therapy, however, there remains a significant number of patients who require surgical intervention.

Before surgical evaluation, a patient with suspected VPI should be evaluated by a speech pathologist. The speech pathologist may measure hypernasality, hyponasality, nasal emission, and articulation in addition to glottal stop, pharyngeal fricatives, or pharyngeal stop. At our institution, a combined examination is performed with nasal endoscopy and speech assessment. During this procedure, an otolaryngologist places the tip of a fiberoptic laryngoscope in the nasopharynx directly above the velopharyngeal sphincter. This allows for direct visualization of the movement of the sphincter. With the sphincter under visualization, the speech pathologist then leads the patient through speech assessments. The nose should be anesthetized with topical lidocaine to improve comfort. Children aged six and above are usually able to tolerate this procedure easily. Younger children can often

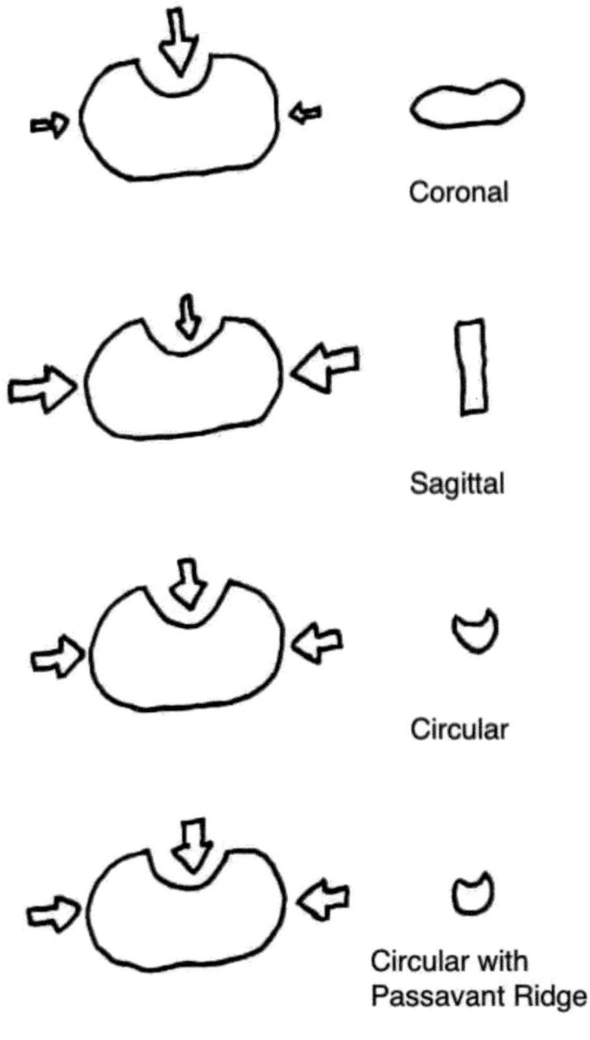

Figure 1.
Velopharynx directional movements of closure patterns.

complete the assessment, but appropriate expectations should be made clear to the parents. Occasionally, assessments may be delayed until the child can successfully cooperate with the exam.

There are four basic closure patterns that the gap is likely to follow: coronal, the most common, in which the movement of the velum closes the velopharyngeal port with little medial motion of the lateral pharyngeal walls; sagittal, the least common, where medial movement of the lateral pharyngeal walls cause closure with minimal velum movement; circular, where both velum and pharyngeal wall movement contribute to velopharyngeal port closure; and circular with the Passavant ridge, which is similar to the circular pattern but with the addition of anterior movement of the posterior pharyngeal wall. A sagittal closure is most common in patients with persistent VPI post-cleft palate repair. Closure pattern is important in determining which surgery will best address the pharyngeal wall motion and control airflow through the port (**Figure 1**).

Magnetic Resonance Imaging (MRI) is also useful in VPI evaluation. While MRIs are noninvasive and may be easier to perform on small children, they do not provide images detailing velopharyngeal motion during speech. Lastly, nasometry measures acoustic activity in the patient's nasal cavity, allowing comparison between the patient's nasalance and normal speech. Nasometry is conducted using a headset with microphones placed in front of the nose and the mouth, separated by a metal plate. Nasometry contributes an objective measure of a patient's nasal acoustic energy to the speech pathologists subjective observations.

3. Assessment of aerodigestive tract anatomy

Prior to the surgical treatment of VPI, an overall assessment of the patient's airway and vasculature must be made. Patients with velocardial syndrome frequently have medialized carotid arteries and assessment via CT angiography is essential in preventing operative complications.

Another preoperative consideration is breathing obstruction. Placement of pharyngeal flaps will obstruct nasal breathing to a degree and may worsen existing breathing difficulties. In cases where the patient already experiences obstruction, a sphincter pharyngoplasty may be better since postoperative breathing obstruction is less than in a posterior pharyngeal flap placement.

Adenoidectomy is often necessary before pharyngoplasty or pharyngeal flap. This is because removal of the adenoids facilitates in raising the pharyngeal flap and in optimizing the pharynx for attachment of the flaps during sphincter pharyngoplasty. If there is tonsillar hypertrophy, tonsillectomy is needed prior to pharyngeal surgery to reduce the risk of developing postoperative sleep apnea. If sphincter pharyngoplasty is planned, the otolaryngologist must take care to preserve the posterior tonsillar pillars so that they can be used for pharyngoplasty flaps.

4. Operative procedures

If the patient presents with sagittal or circular closure is present, a superiorly based pharyngeal flap is recommended. If the closure pattern is coronal relatively small to intermediate in size, a sphincter pharyngoplasty will restore port function. The Furlow palatoplasty is chosen if the closure pattern is coronal with a small gap. In this case, the surgeon may feel that VPI will be addressed with the soft palate lengthening achieved by this technique. A detailed description of each surgical approach can be found below [4].

4.1 Furlow palatoplasty (double opposing Z-palatoplasty)

Furlow double opposing z-palatoplasty is a technique to repair cleft palate. The procedure lengthens the soft palate and is called a "Z-plasty" because of the Z shaped scar that remains. A Dingman retractor is first placed and the palate injected with epinephrine. For a submucous cleft, the procedure begins with dividing the soft palate anteriorly along the midline to approximately 3 mm posterior to the hard palate junction (**Figure 2**).

For an incomplete soft palate cleft, the incision first traverses along the free margin of the soft palate in an axial plane. Next, the tips and medial edges of the uvula are trimmed. A posteriorly based myomucosal flap is incised and elevated on the left side, and an anteriorly based myomucosal flap is then elevated on the right to create a Z-shaped incision. The left-sided muscle and oral mucosa are raised from the nasal mucosa by separating the muscle from the hard palate. On the right, only the mucosa and the submucosa are raised, leaving muscle on the nasal mucosa. The nasal side midline is also divided once both palatal flaps are raised [5] (**Figure 3**).

Incisions are made on the newly formed nasal flaps in a mirror image to the oral flaps. The right-sided nasal myomucosal flap must be rotated posteriorly, and the left-sided mucosal flaps anteriorly. The nasal side is closed first using 4–0 absorbable sutures starting at the apices of the flaps, then at their horizontal midlines, then finishing on the anterior and posterior flap edges (**Figure 4**).

Once the nasal flaps are secured, the oral flaps are transposed and closed using 4–0 absorbable sutures except at the midline, where durable 4–0 PDS sutures can reinforce the soft tissues together. Lastly, the uvula must be closed with a horizontal mattress suture (**Figure 5**) [6].

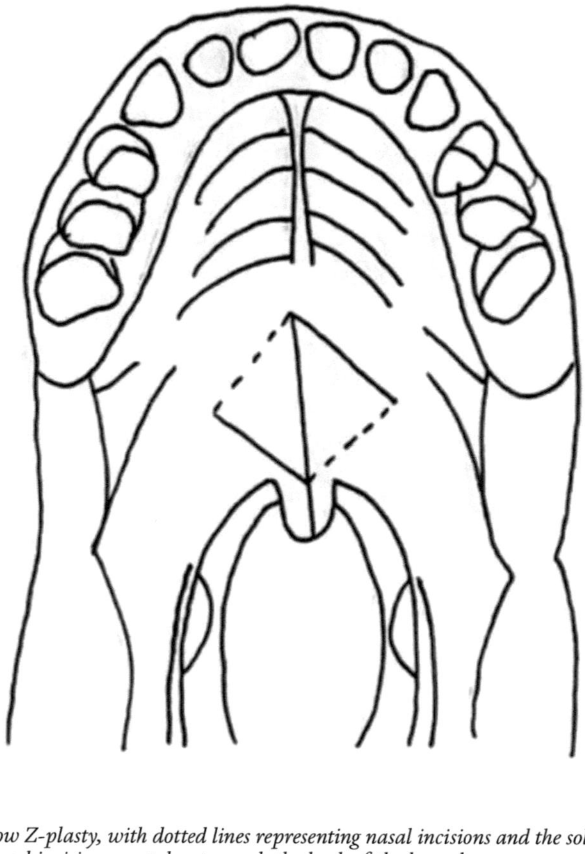

Figure 2.
Incision lines for Furlow Z-plasty, with dotted lines representing nasal incisions and the solid lines representing oral incisions. The lateral incisions are taken towards the hook of the hamulus.

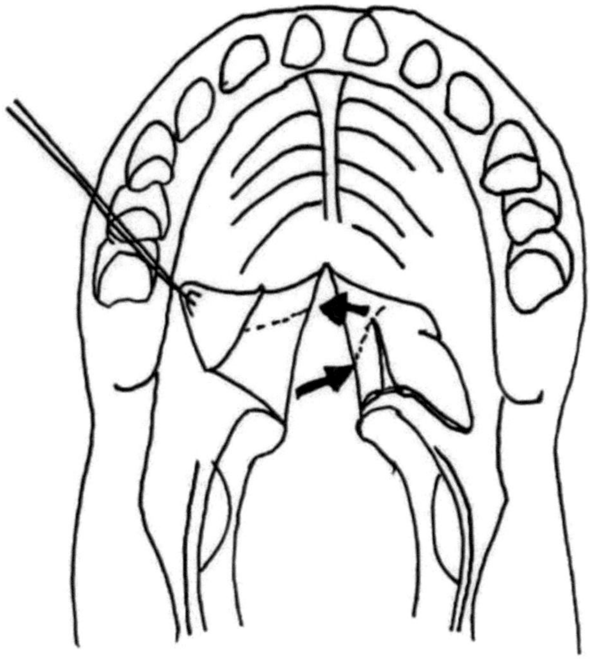

Figure 3.
Raised oral flaps reveal nasal incision lines, which mirror the shape and angle of their opposing oral flaps. Arrows indicate where the nasal tissue will lay between the incised nasal flaps.

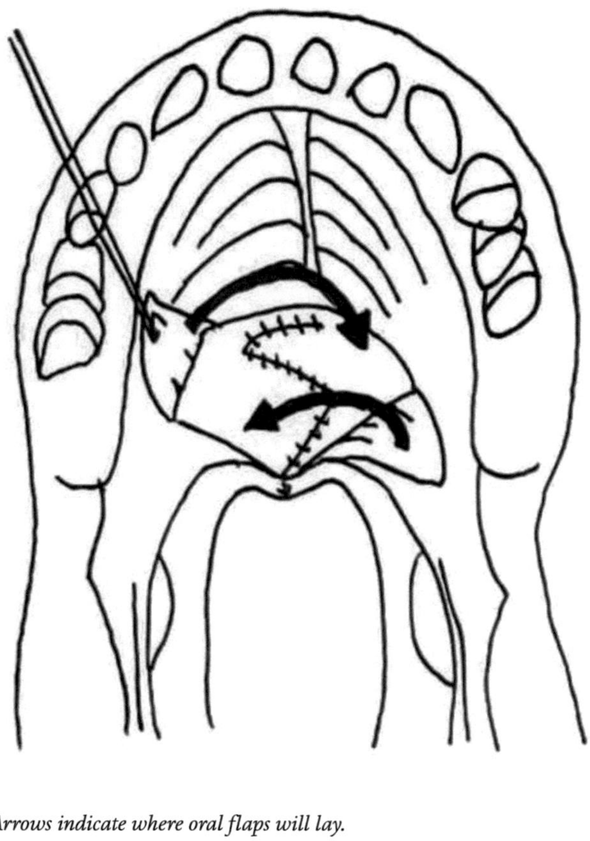

Figure 4.
Secured nasal flaps. Arrows indicate where oral flaps will lay.

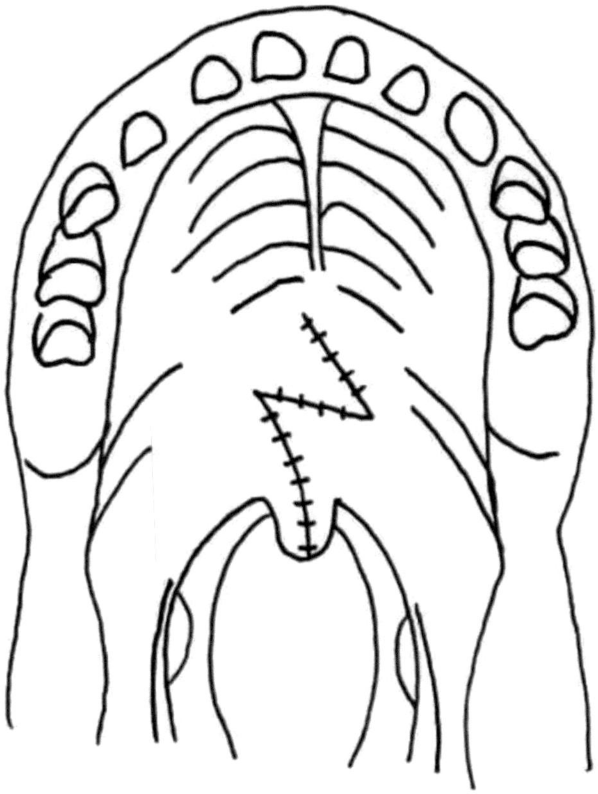

Figure 5.
Suture pattern for final closure of the Furlow Z-plasty.

4.2 Pharyngeal flap

The Pharyngeal flap is the most common secondary surgical procedure used to treat VPI. It involves attaching tissue from the posterior pharyngeal wall to the soft palate creating a partial obstruction of the nasal and oral cavities save for two small laeral ports. The surgery works most effectively on patients with sagittal or circular closure patterns because these patterns retain sufficient lateral wall movement. First, the soft palate is incised along the oral midline from the uvula to the soft-hard palate junction (**Figure 6**).

A "book flap" incision is also made on the posterior pharyngeal wall to the prevertebral fascia. This fascial layer is easily identified by its white appearance and relative lack of vascularity. A submucosal pharyngeal flap is elevated superiorly while the two mucosal flaps are lifted laterally. The free inferior edge of the submucosal flap is then sutured to the posterior nasal edge of the soft palate (**Figure 7**).

The book flap incision is closed by simple approximation of the pharyngeal mucosa. The two oral soft palate flaps are sutured to the base of the pharyngeal submucosal flap and to each other to hide the pharyngeal flap (**Figures 8** and **9**).

VPI closures may be conducted via a superiorly based pharyngeal flap [7].

4.3 Sphincter pharyngoplasty

Sphincter pharyngoplasty is best suited for patients with poor posterior pharyngeal movement and small velopharyngeal ports. The surgery narrows the nasal orifice, limiting nasal airflow during speech. In contrast to pharyngeal flaps, pharyngoplasty narrows the central nasal orifice without creating velopharyngeal ports [8].

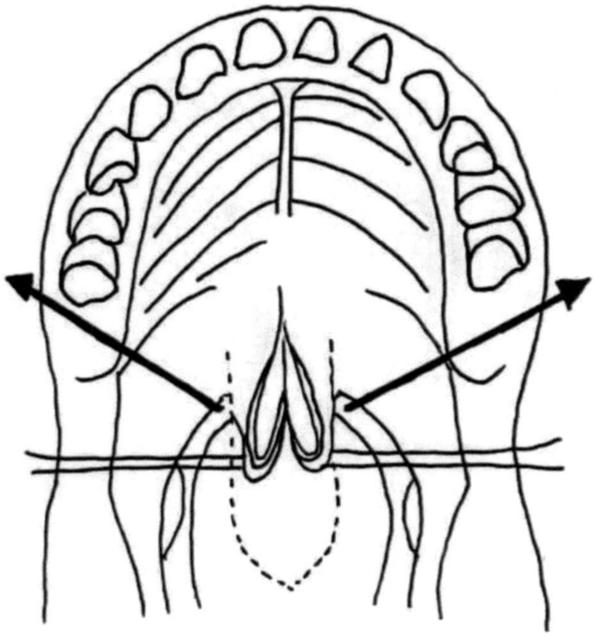

Figure 6.
Midline incision divides soft palate to posterior nasal spine. Arrows indicate the direction that the incised uvula will be lifted in preparation for the next step.

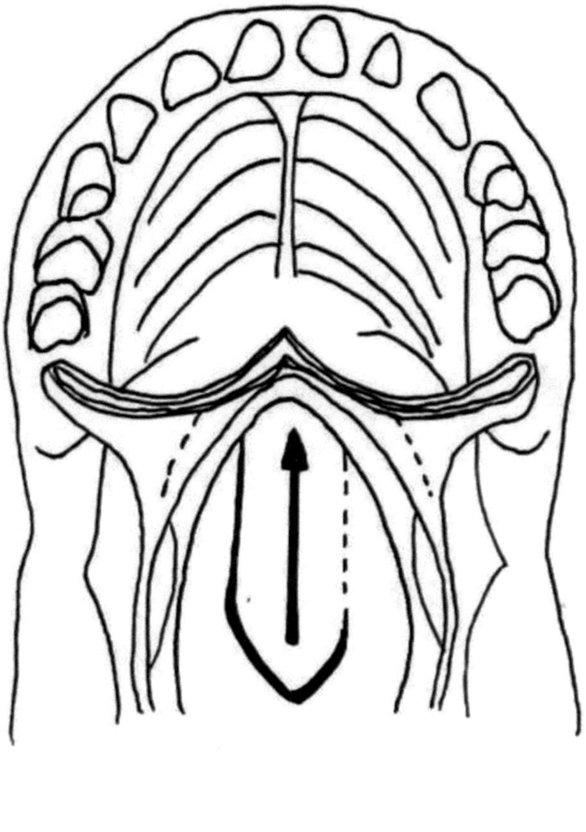

Figure 7.
Book flap incision along the dotted line on the posterior pharyngeal wall that will line lateral ports with mucous membrane. Arrow indicates where the book flap will be raised and secured.

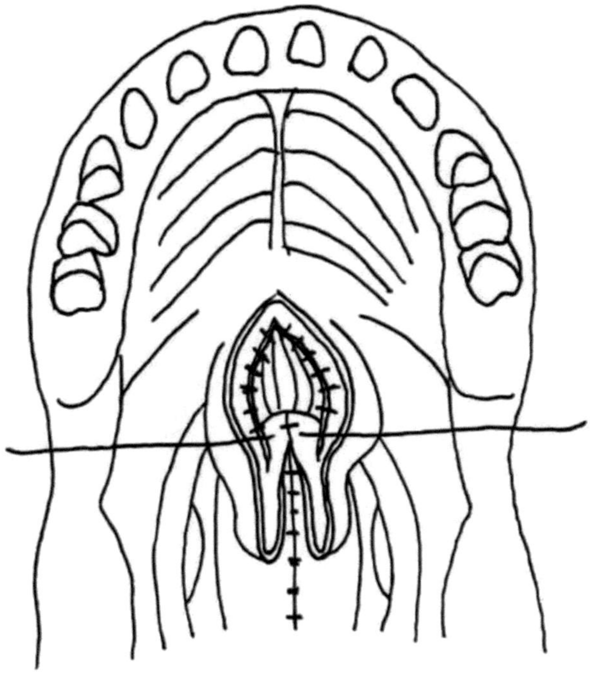

Figure 8.
Two soft palate flaps used to cover raw tissue of pharyngeal flap are sutured to pharyngeal flap base.

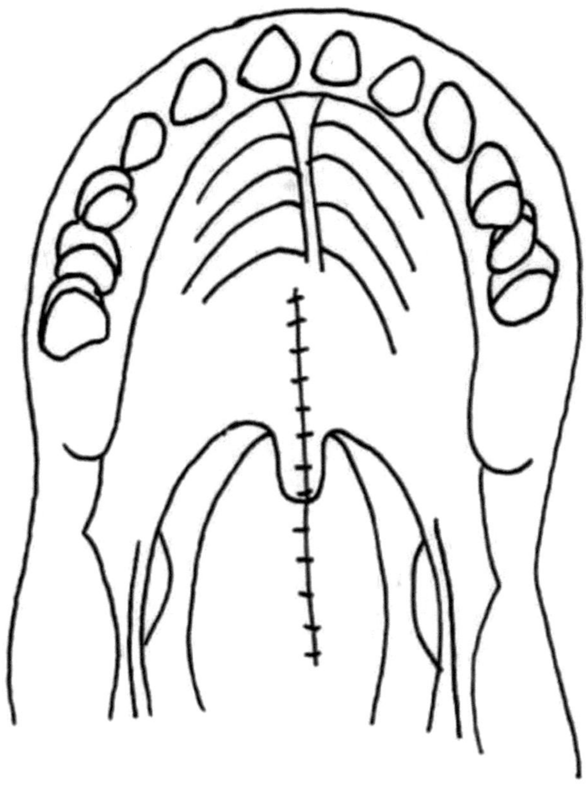

Figure 9.
Closure pattern following pharyngeal flap placement.

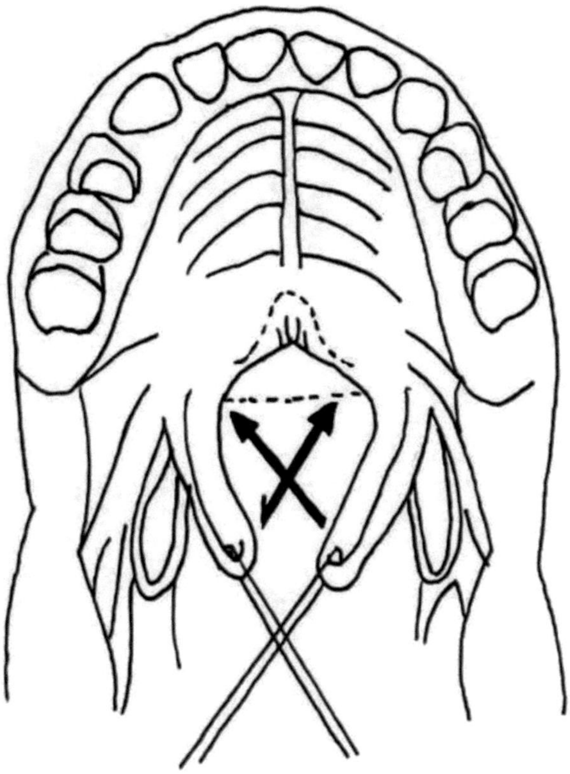

Figure 10.
Raising of both tonsillar pillar flaps. Arrows indicate that the flaps will be laid in a criss-cross fashion.

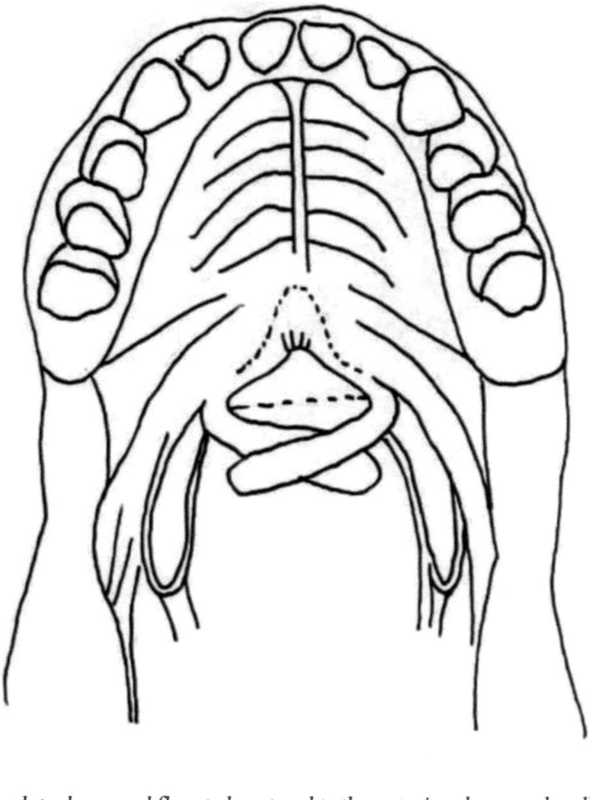

Figure 11.
Ready position of the palatopharyngeal flaps to be sutured to the posterior pharyngeal wall.

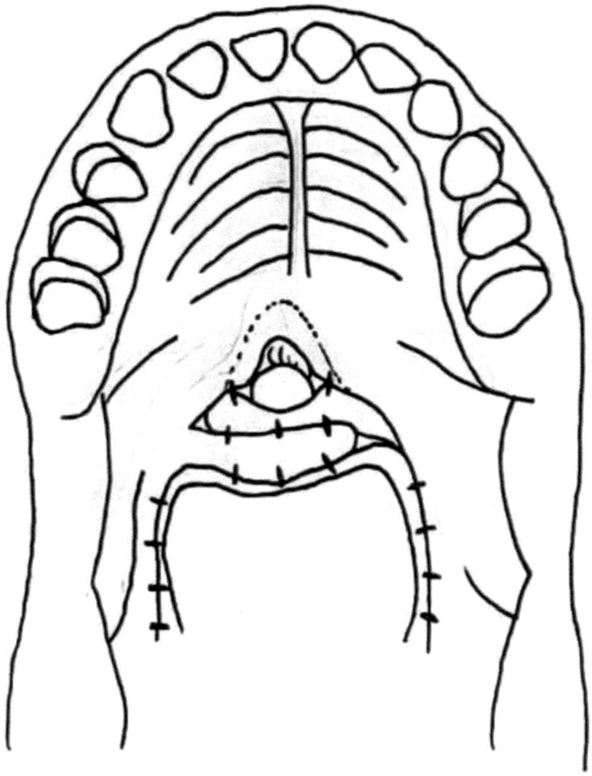

Figure 12.
Completed sphincter pharyngoplasty.

The procedure begins with a rubber catheter that is inserted into the nose and sutured to the uvula to expose the posterior pharyngeal wall. Next, after raising the myomucosal flaps, the posterior pharyngeal wall is incised transversely (**Figure 10**).

The cut should extend from the posterior limb of one of the lateral flaps to the other. Donor sites are closed with 4–0 polyglactin sutures then the catheter is removed before closing. The left flap's superior mucosa is sutured to the posterior pharyngeal wall's superior incision. Then the left flap's caudal mucosa is sutured to the right flap's superior mucosa, causing the flaps to overlap. The right flap's causal mucosa is sutured to the pharyngeal wall's posterior mucosa (**Figure 11**).

The lateral flaps are sutured together in position to secure the new sphincter. The ideal diameter of the resulting port should be one centimeter (**Figure 12**).

5. Recovery

The procedure time for Furlow double opposing Z-palatoplasty is approximately 1.5 hours. Post-operative time spent in the hospitalis most likely one day. For a few days, pain will be minimal to moderate and can be managed with oral medications. The patient should eat only soft foods for 5–7 days after the operation. The palatal wound takes 3–4 weeks to heal, and restraints may be needed to keep the patient from disrupting the incision area [1]. Complications from this procedure include flap breakdown or shrinkage. Additionally, the patient may develop obstructive sleep apnea or nasal congestion. Although the surgery improves speech, speech therapy is recommended to correct post-operatively learnt errors. With surgery and therapy, the speech normalization rate is approximately 60–70%. Refractory cases may require pharyngeal flaps or pharyngoplasty.

For secondary surgeries like pharyngeal flap and sphincter palatoplasty, patients are monitored overnight and may begin a soft or liquid diet that same day. The patient should sleep with their head elevated for two weeks postoperatively. Any required speech therapy may resume after their three week follow-up. A post-surgery velopharyngeal inspection will occur 3 and 12 months after surgery.

6. Conclusion

Choice of surgical approach to treat VPI depends on the patient's individual anatomy as well as severity. Therefore, evaluation prior to surgery is important in a surgeon's decision of what approach they will use. Due to possible complications and risks involving important arteries, airway obstruction, and future speech ability, a surgeon should carefully consider the procedures above and their respective risks and benefits before operating. Each possible surgery (the Furlow Double Opposing Z-Palatoplasty, sphincter pharyngoplasty, posterior pharyngeal wall injection, and a pharyngeal flap pharyngoplasty) has its own set of conditions under which the patient will experience maximum results in correcting hypernasality, nasal emissions, nasal regurgitation of food and liquid and communication difficulties. The assessment and procedure descriptions above should be sufficient information for a surgeon to choose what approach is best, as well as provide adequate background information on VPI.

Author details

Nguyen Pham[1,2*] and Isabella Rodoni[3]

1 University of California Irvine School of Medicine, Irvine, CA, United States

2 Children's Hospital of Orange County, Orange, CA, United States

3 Cornell University, Ithaca, NY, United States

*Address all correspondence to: nspham@gmail.com

References

[1] T.A. Emara, M.D., A.S Quriba, M.D., "Posterior Pharyngeal Flap for Velopharyngeal Insufficiency Patients: A New Technique for Flap Inset," *The Laryngoscope,* 122:2 pg.260-65, (2012).

[2] A. Evans, T. Driscoll, B. Ackermann, "Prevalence of velopharyngeal insufficiency in woodwind and brass students," *Occupational Medicine*, 61:480-482, (2011).

[3] P.K. Patel, M.D., "Surgical Treatment of Velopharyngeal Dysfunction," *eMedicine*, (2018).

[4] K. Nagy, G. Swennen, "Oral Mucosal Z-Plasty in Combination with Intravelar Veloplasty," *Plastic and Reconstructive Surgery Global Open,* 3:7, (2015).

[5] E. Gunther, J.R. Wisser, M.A. Cohen, and A. S. Brown, "Palatoplasty: Furlow's Double Reversing Z-Plasty versus Intravelar Veloplasty," *The Cleft Palate-Craniofacial Journal: Official Publication of the American Cleft Palate-Craniofacial Association,* 35:6 pg.546-49, (1998).

[6] C. Havstam, A. Lohmander, et al., "Evaluation of VPI-Assessment with Videofluoroscopy and Nasoendoscopy," *British Journal of Plastic Surgery,* 58:7 pg. 922-31, (2005).

[7] S.M. Nam, "Surgical Treatment of Velopharyngeal Insufficiency," *Archives of Craniofacial Surgery,* 19:3 pg.163-67, (2018).

[8] N. Raol, C.J. Hartnick, "Sphincter Pharyngoplasty," *Surgery for Pediatric Velopharyngeal Insufficiency,* 76:58-66, (2015).

Chapter 7

Diagnosis and Management of Obstructive Sleep Apnea

Ho-Hyun (Brian) Sun and Sally Sun

Abstract

Obstructive sleep apnea (OSA) represents a major public health issue affecting over 10% of the general adult, more than 80% of the geriatric, and up to 11% of the pediatric populations. Numerous studies have demonstrated distinct associations between OSA and diabetes, daytime drowsiness, and cardiopulmonary compromise including myocardial infarction. Considering the estimated rate of underdiagnosis, OSA is expected to exert a significant unrealized toll on the global healthcare infrastructure with the number of diagnoses increasing each year. The diagnosis of OSA entails subjective and objective evaluations including sleep surveys and polysomnography. Accordingly, treatment of OSA also encompasses a large variety of conservative, pharmacologic, and surgical interventions. Treatment selection remains a difficult but critical part of intervention especially when multiple modalities are required. This chapter aims to describe not only the presentation of this head and neck airway pathology but the interprofessional management strategies employed.

Keywords: polysomnography, apnea, hypopnea, obstructive sleep apnea, obesity, continuous positive airway pressure, septoplasty, uvulopalatopharyngoplasty, hyoid suspension, genioglossus advancement, maxillomandibular advancement, hypoglossal nerve stimulation

1. Introduction

Obstructive sleep apnea (OSA) is a common disease of the head and neck respiratory tract with severe systemic ramifications [1, 2]. It is characterized by multiple episodes of apnea or hypopnea during sleep resulting from partial and/or complete collapse of the upper airway [3].

OSA affects 10% or more of the population with males at increasingly greater risk than females [4]. It contributes to chronic conditions such as obesity, diabetes, myocardial infarction, and daytime drowsiness that leads to frequent motor vehicle accidents [3]. Many surgical and non-surgical treatment modalities exist, including continuous positive air pressure (CPAP) devices that keep the patency of the airway via exerting a baseline artificial inspiratory pressure. When patients are unable or unwilling to tolerate these bulky fixtures, they often require surgery to mechanically increase their airway volume [5].

Studies have described factors associated with the presentation and severity of OSA. Conditions that narrow the upper airway are particularly injurious to the at-risk patient. Physiologic features such as obesity (which increases the mass of the soft tissues around the neck), decreases in muscle or neural tone (which frequently results from sedation or old age), congenital gnathic hypoplasias (which may exist without other notable medical findings), and craniofacial syndromes (which could contribute to abnormal hypoplasia of multiple craniofacial features) have been implicated [6].

2. History

Ancient Greeks first noted OSA or OSA-like snoring conditions in their 4th century BC accounts of Dionysius, the tyrant of Heraclea who was said to be "obese beyond measure." The first modern medical description is attributed to James Russell and his peers as a syndrome of obesity and daytime drowsiness. OSA was poetically if not erroneously named the "Pickwickian syndrome" after the snoring "fat boy Joe" in Charles Dickens's novel "The Posthumous Papers of the Pickwick Club." [7] Dickens's tale would depict the life of an obese servant boy whose daytime activities were marred by debilitating drowsiness as often noted in modern OSA patients.

While clinicians and writers alike noted the distinct obesity of most OSA patients, obstruction was deemed inevitable until the development of the CPAP device in 1981 by Colin Sullivan and colleagues at the University of Sydney [8]. CPAP first saw use as a bulky nasal device that soon became the gold standard in OSA care.

3. Causes

OSA frequently co-presents with chronic conditions, the most prevalent of which is obesity. Obesity increases the mass and volume of parapharyngeal tissues, which can fall back in a supine position to cause respiratory obstruction during sleep. In fact, supine sleepers and patients with adeno-tonsillar enlargements experience OSA more frequently [9]. Metabolic conditions like hyperlipidemia and diabetes that may result from one or both of OSA and obesity [10].

Similarly, other pathoses leading to airway narrowing also predispose patients to OSA. Central and peripheral neural injuries that decrease the airway muscle tone have been shown to contribute to OSA in patients suffering from trauma [11]. Craniofacial syndromes like Down Syndrome that cause retrolingual hyperplasia and/or mandibular hypoplasia have been implicated in higher instances of OSA [6]. As such, OSA may also entail a genetic component with shared genes involving the formation of the nose, mouth, and throat likely predisposing certain families to higher rates of disease.

4. Signs and symptoms

As noted above, OSA has historically been defined by daytime drowsiness, loud snoring, and nighttime choking. This frequently leads to a higher incidence of automotive accidents and narcolepsy-like episodes [4]. Furthermore, implications in neurocognitive pathoses including impairments to attention, executive functioning, and long-term memory have been documented [12].

More recent studies indicate that OSA may also be an etiological factor behind diabetes, hypertension, coronary artery disease, and stroke. Appropriate treatment of OSA may reduce the risk of developing these conditions [10]. Obesity may also play a role as both a risk factor and a complication of OSA. Studies stipulate that alterations of molecular signaling pathways via repeated hypoxic episodes contribute to autonomic dysregulation, systemic inflammation, cardiopulmonary irregularities, and organic oxidation which predispose patients to metabolic diseases [13]. In fact, OSA has been linked to an increased risk of early death in patients under the age of 70 [2].

Studies of OSA in children are less common and may be confounded by the effects of puberty. They nonetheless indicate that while children with sleep-disordered breathing are at risk of attention and executive deficits like their adult counterparts, they show additional deficits in empathy, social behaviors, and phonological processing [12]. Children with OSA may also be predisposed to pulmonary hypertension and nocturnal enuresis [14].

5. Diagnosis

Today, polysomnography plays a central role in the diagnosis of both central and obstructive sleep apnea. A patient's apnea-hypopnea index (AHI) is taken along with the patient's brain (electroencephalography or EEG), eye (electrooculography or EOG), muscle (electromyography or EMG), and/or heart (electrocardiography or ECG) activities which enumerates the average number of apneic or hypopneic events per hour of physiologic sleep. An apneic event is defined as a 90% or more reduction of airflow lasting at least 10 seconds. An hypopneic event is defined as a 30–90% reduction of airflow lasting at least 10 seconds accompanied by a 3% or greater decrease in pulse oxygenation [15]. A diagnosis of mild OSA is made with an AHI of 5 to 15, moderate OSA with AHI of 15 to 30, and severe OSA with AHI of 30 or more events per hour (**Table 1**). Significant ECG abnormalities may also be present, which could indicate an increased severity of disease [13]. This scale is adjusted for the categorization of OSA in children. Pediatric OSA is classified as mild if AHI is between 1 to 5, moderate if between 5 to 10, and severe if greater than 10 events per hour.

Though less common, some literature instead utilize the respiratory disturbance index (RDI) to diagnose or monitor the progress of OSA. The RDI is determined as a sum of AHI and respiratory-effort related arousals (RERAs), which are characterized by increasing respiratory effort for 10 seconds or more leading to an arousal from sleep. Similarly to the AHI scale, the American Academy of Sleep Medicine regards RDI of 5 to 15 as mild, 15 to 30 as moderate, and more than 30 as severe [16].

Drug-induced sleep endoscopy (DISE) is another diagnostic modality for the detection of upper airway collapse during sleep. A sedative agent such as propofol,

AHI or RDI	OSA Severity
Less than 5	None
5 to 14	Mild
15 to 29	Moderate
More than 30	Severe

Table 1.
AHI and RDI scales [13, 15, 16].

How likely are you to doze off or fall asleep in the following scenarios?	
0 = Never	
1 = Slight chance of dozing off	
2 = Moderate chance of dozing off	
3 = High chance of dozing off	
Total Score – A score of greater than 10 denotes a higher risk of OSA	
0 – 5: Lower normal daytime sleepiness	
6 – 10: Higher normal daytime sleepiness	
11 – 12: Mild excessive daytime sleepiness	
13 – 15: Moderate excessive daytime sleepiness	
16 – 24: Severe excessive daytime sleepiness	
Scenario	Score
Sitting and reading	_______
Watching TV	_______
Sitting inactive in a public place (i.e. theater)	_______
As a passenger in a car for an hour	_______
Lying down to rest in the afternoon	_______
Sitting and talking to someone	_______
Sitting quietly after lunch without alcohol	_______
While stopped in traffic for a few minutes	_______

Table 2.
Epworth Sleepiness Scale [18].

Item 1: if "Yes," a point is added.	
Item 2: if "c" or "d," a point is added	
Item 3: if "a" or "b," a point is added	
Item 4: if "a," a point is added	
Item 5: if "a" or "b," two points are added.	
Category 1 is "positive" if the total points above are 2 or higher.	
Item 6: if "a" or "b," a point is added	
Item 7: if "a" or "b," a point is added	
Item 8: if "a," a point is added	
Category 2 is "positive" if the total points above are 2 or higher.	
Category 3 is "positive" if the answer to item 10 is "Yes" or if the patient BMI is greater than 30kg/m^2	
Patients are considered high risk of 2 or more categories are deemed positive.	
Item 1: Do you snore?	**Item 6**: How often do you feel tired or fatigued after sleep?
A. Yes	A. Nearly every day
B. No	B. 3-4 times per week
C. Do not know	C. 1-2 times per week
	D. 1-2 times per month
	E. Never or nearly never

Item 2: Your snoring is	**Item 7:** During your waking time, do you feel tired or fatigued?
A. Slightly louder than breathing.	A. Nearly every day
B. As loud as talking	B. 3-4 times per week
C. Louder than talking	C. 1-2 times per week
D. Can be heard in adjacent rooms	D. 1-2 times per month
E. I do not snore	E. Never or nearly never
Item 3: How often do you snore?	**Item 8:** Have you ever nodded off or fallen asleep while driving a vehicle?
A. Nearly every day	A. Yes
B. 3-4 times per week	B. No
C. 1-2 times per week	
D. 1-2 times per month	
E. Never or nearly never	
Item 4: Has your snoring ever bothered other people?	**Item 9:** How often do you nod off while driving?
A. Yes	A. Nearly every day
B. No	B. 3-4 times per week
C. Do not know	C. 1-2 times per week
	D. 1-2 times per month
	E. Never or nearly never
Item 5: Has anyone noticed that you stop breathing during sleep?	**Item 10:** Do you have high blood pressure?
A. Nearly every day	A. Yes
B. 3-4 times per week	B. No
C. 1-2 times per week	C. Do not know
D. 1-2 times per month	
E. Never or nearly never	

Table 3.
Berlin Questionnaire [19].

midazolam, or dexmedetomidine is administered to create a somewhat artificial state of sleep, during which a flexible endoscope is utilized to view the nasopharyngeal and oropharyngeal airways to monitor areas of collapse. While DISE can be a useful modality in detecting the degree and pattern of obstruction, its use may be limited as a result of 1) unnatural sleep patterns as a result of drug-induced nature of the slumber, 2) difficulty of maintaining the appropriate degree of sedation without causing undue cessation of respiration, and 3) uncertain reproducibility when scoring the degree of obstruction across different observers [17]. The use of propofol and/or dexmedetomidine purportedly re-creates a more natural pattern of sleep when compared to other medications like benzodiazepines.

The clinical manifestation of daytime sleepiness can be monitored via several patient surveys such as the Berlin and Epworth Sleepiness questionnaires (**Tables 2** and **3**). Recent studies suggest that the STOP-BANG questionnaire (**Table 4**) as devised by researchers at the University of Toronto is particularly effective not only as a screening tool but also as an adjunct to clinical follow up after operative interventions [21, 22].

A point is added for each question that is answered with a "yes."
Snoring: Do you snore loudly?
Tired: Do you often feel tired, fatigued, or sleepy during the daytime?
Observed choking: Has anyone observed you choking during sleep?
Pressure: Do you have or are being treated for high blood pressure?
Body mass index: Is your BMI more than 35kg/m^2?
Age: Are you older than 50 years of age?
Neck size: Is your shirt collar size >17 in for males or >16 in for females?
Gender: Are you biologically male?
In general, patients with a score of 2 or below are considered low risk, 3 to 4 intermediate risk, and 5 or greater high risk.

Table 4.
STOP-BANG Questionnaire [20].

In general, patients with a score of 2 or below are considered low risk, 3 to 4 intermediate risk, and 5 or greater high risk.

6. Management

Treatment of OSA may frequently reverse its systemic consequences, though permanent brain alterations may occur that prevent complete recovery of deficits in psychomotor functioning [12]. However, most studies concur that metabolic consequences (including those associated with diabetes and obesity) improve after resolution or improvement of OSA [4, 6, 12].

An effective management of OSA can be categorized as either a "success" or a "cure." In general, a successful treatment denotes a 50% or greater reduction in AHI such that it decreases to an AHI of 20 events per hour or less. The definition of a curative treatment is more stringent and requires the reduction of AHI to 5 events s per hour or less [13]. Interventional success may also be defined as a 50% or greater reduction in RDI with a post-procedural RDI of 15 or less [23].

7. Conservative management

Conservative therapy remains the mainstay of OSA treatment because of their low risk and reversibility of treatment. Furthermore, pharmacologic and/or surgical interventions may require a stricter set of inclusion criteria and may not be appropriate for every patient [24].

Conservative therapy can be as non-invasive as a simple avoidance of certain substances or dietary patterns. As described previously, avoidance of obesity via healthy diet and possibly even exercise alone may improve symptoms of OSA [25]. Abstinence from sedating compounds and airway muscle relaxants – such as alcohol - is also beneficial [26]. Patients should cease exposure to airway irritants like tobacco smoke and partake in activities that encourage patency of the airway like sleeping in inclined or lateral positions and playing wind instruments [26–29].

CPAP devices are considered the gold standard of OSA therapy. They function by creating consistent air pressures in airways to keep them patent during sleep. CPAP has a long history of demonstrated efficacy, and its use has also been associated with decreases in a number of associated conditions including cognitive impairment, daytime drowsiness, and cardiovascular disease [30–32]. CPAP machines are nonetheless bulky and uncomfortable to wear, leading to a high rate of noncompliance [33]. Modified equipment such as bilevel positive airway pressure (BiPAP) or automatically-titrated (APAP) devices, which monitors breathing to exert a higher pressure during inhalation and a lower pressure during exhalation, can reduce discomfort associated with their use [34].

Oral appliance therapy is also considered an acceptable, reversible therapy for OSA especially in cases of mild or moderate sleep apnea [35]. The devices typically function by inducing an anterior posture of the mandible that, in theory, helps increase the antero-posterior diameter of the retrolingual airway. While oral appliances are much more compact and often better tolerated, its efficacy remains controversial and long term use may be associated with dry mouth, dental trauma, and jaw pain [26, 36].

8. Pharmacologic interventions

In general, the evidence supporting pharmacotherapy remains insufficient. [24, 37] Antidepressants and serotonin-promoting compounds were studied because activation of serotonin 5-HT_2 receptors in the brainstem was shown to induce excitatory input to the hypoglossal neurons, which in turn incites an anterior advancement of the tongue [38]. Mirtazapine in particular was shown to reduce AHI in the short term, but its long-term administration is associated with sedation and weight gain, which are known adverse risk factors of worsening OSA [39]. Paroxetine was also studied but its effects were found not to be significant, [40] possibly because non-discriminatory activation of both peripheral 5-HT_3 and 5-HT_2 and receptors has been associated with REM-associated apnea [41].

Parasympathomimetics like donepezil may modulate airway and/or tongue muscle contraction via cholinergic pathways. Its use was associated with a reduction in AHI by approximately 20%, [42] which would not meet the clinical definition of successful or curative treatment in all but mild cases. Respiratory smooth-muscle relaxants like theophylline were found to be either ineffective or to trigger counter-productive deteriorations in sleep quality because of their stimulatory properties [43].

Dronabinol and a combination of ondansetron and fluoxetine demonstrated some promise in controlling the rate of AHI in sleep apneic patients. While ondansetron or fluoxetine alone were ineffective, their combination showed more than a 40% reduction in AHI. Investigators stipulate that fluoxetine may stimulate central 5-HT_2 receptors while ondansetron suppresses the activation of their peripheral 5-HT_3 counterparts [44]. Dronabinol also incurred dose-dependent 40–50% reductions in AHI over a 6-week period of use. Cannabinoids like dronabinol activates cannabinoid type 1 (CB1) receptors, which in turn also antagonizes the actions of 5-HT_3 receptors [45]. However, neither the ondansetron-fluoxetine combination nor dronabinol showed clear clinical improvements in daytime drowsiness.

9. Sleep surgery

While conservative therapy is considered the first line intervention for OSA, surgery may be indicated in patients who are unable or unwilling to tolerate lifelong conservative therapy [5]. A 2004 study of military veterans suggested that even singular surgical therapy may provide more than a 30% increase in overall survival benefit [46]. In fact, a combination of multiple surgical modalities may achieve a 60% reduction in AHI, which is comparable to that of CPAP which demonstrates between a 60 to 70% reduction [47, 48].

10. Tonsillectomy

Surgical intervention may encompass the soft and/or the hard tissues of the upper airway. Tonsillectomy is a soft tissue-oriented procedure that may be of benefit especially in children since their apneic episodes are predominantly caused by enlarged lymphoid tissues of the upper airway [3]. The long-term efficacy, however, is not yet well established [49]. In tonsillectomy, the lymphoid tissues and its capsular container are dissected wholly from its surrounding tissues. Sharp dissection with scalpel and electro- or diathermic-cautery may be used, followed by blunt dissection [50]. Notable vessels in the area are ligated using sutures which may be assisted by using topical thrombin. Post-operative bleeding may be significant which manifests in approximately 2% of patients and typically occurs approximately 1 to 2 weeks post-operatively [51].

11. Septoplasty with or without turbinate reduction

Septoplasty may also be conducted to address obstructions of the nasal passageway, which could worsen OSA symptoms. It is frequently conducted in patients with or without OSA to help relieve internal nasal valve obstruction. While nasal surgery alone may not significantly reduce AHI, it may be a viable adjunct therapy when utilized with another intervention [52]. Septoplasty with turbinate reduction has been associated with better tolerance of CPAP therapy [53].

To conduct septoplasty, an intranasal vertical incision is made through the septal mucosa and the perichondrium on the side of the obstruction (**Figure 1**). The approach is then taken posteriorly in a sub-perichondral fashion using a blunt instrument. The overlying soft tissues are carefully dissected from the obstructing spur or deviation to avoid tears. Vertical chondrotomies are made anterior and posterior to the obstruction so that the mucosa may be detached from the contralateral septal surface. A horziontal chodrontomy is made connecting the superior edges of the vertical chondrotomies. The horizontal chondrotomy is made at least 1 cm from the superior margin of the septum to preserve the structural integrity of the septum and prevent a saddle defect. The portion of cartilage containing the spur or deviation is then freed from the nasal spine and removed.

Adjunctive turbinate reduction may be accomplished via another vertical, full-thickness incision anterior to the inferior turbinate (or concha) at the attachment point to the lateral nasal wall (**Figure 2**). A subperiosteal plane is raised to expose the osseous turbinate. Forceps may then be introduced through the incision to remove the turbinate in small pieces. The overlying mucosa should also be reduced using a microdebrider without perforating through the soft tissue. Any remaining osseous portions may then be outfractured with a blunt instrument by applying lateral pressure.

The septal and/or turbinate mucosal incisions are sutured closed using a resorbable suture. Doyle splints or multiple interrupted transseptal sutures may be placed for five days to prevent the formation of a septal hematoma.

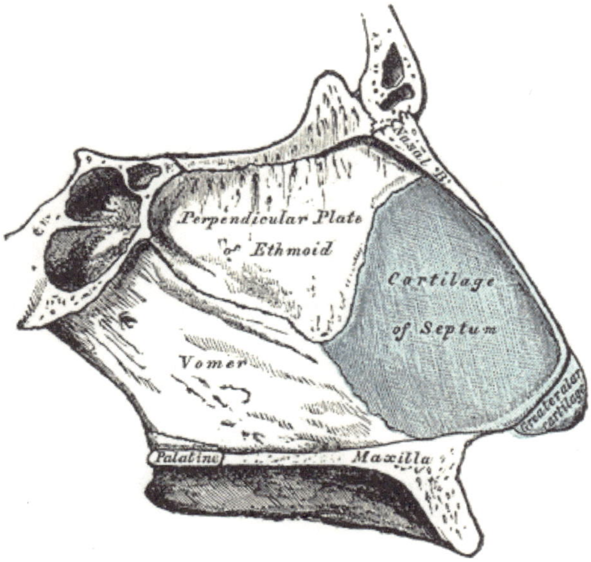

Figure 1.
The cartilaginous septum.

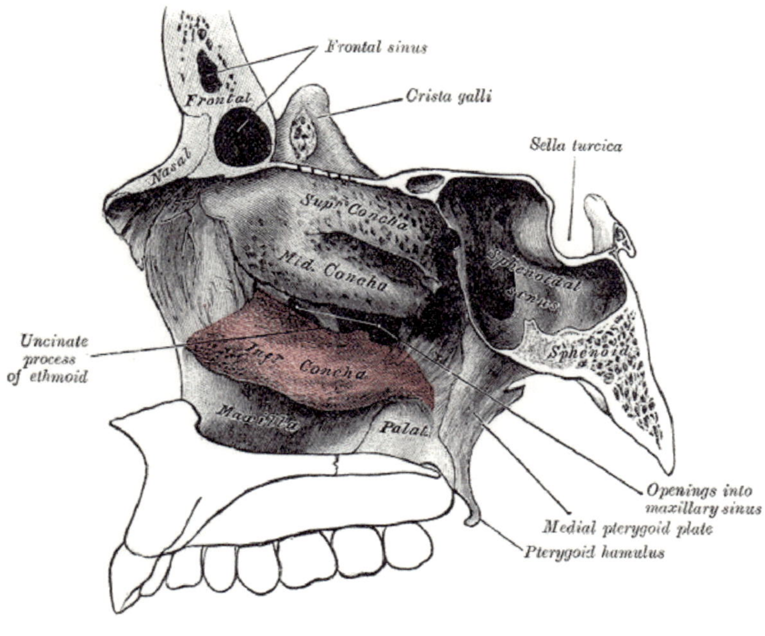

Figure 2.
Inferior turbinate position in the nasal cavity.

12. Uvulopalatopharyngoplasty

Uvulopalatopharyngoplasty (UPPP) is perhaps the most performed sleep surgery. While the large variety of OSA-associated factors make it difficult to gauge the exact success rate of UPPP, it appears to be more efficacious in patients without excessive neck size or BMI. UPPP is also notably less effective in those with multi-level obstructions beyond those of the retropalatal and retrolingual tissues [54].

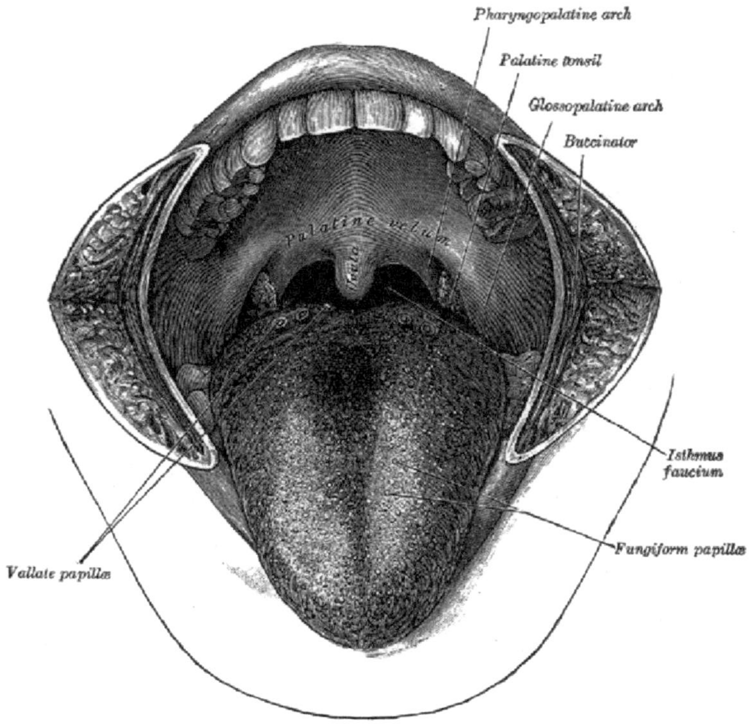

Figure 3.
An anatomic depiction of the uvula, tonsils, and their surrounding pillars.

In UPPP, the uvula, tonsils, and sometimes adenoids are first removed to remove the protrusive bulks of oropharyngeal tissue with particular attention towards preserving the posterior tonsillar pillars (**Figure 3**). The uvula may be excised with a wedge incision through its base to aid in closure.

The operator could then elect to further widen the lateral soft tissues of the oropharynx via lateral expansion pharyngoplasty. The bilateral palatopharyngeus muscles are located through the tonsillectomy incisions, dissected from the pharyngeal walls, then transected at a point approximately 2/3rds of the way from the palate to the tonsillar pillar base. The freed muscles may then be folded antero-superiorly through a tunnel deep to the palatal mucosa or through an incision placed through the palatal soft tissues. The previously transected edge of the palatopharyngeus is then sutured to the fixed aponeurotic tissues around the hamulis such that the action of the palatopharyngeus triggers a lateral expansion of the airway at the soft palate.

The posterior palatal pillars may then be suspended anteriorly via suturing the pillars to the pterygomandibular raphe. The incision sites for the uvula, tonsils, adenoids, and/or palatopharyngeus are sutured closed to create a smooth mucosal surface.

13. Hyoid suspension

Hyoid suspension (HS) is a relatively noninvasive surgical procedure that is commonly performed in conjunction with UPPP or genioglossus advancement. Like UPPP, HS is indicated for milder cases of OSA with retrolingual and hypopharyngeal (not retropalatal) obstructions [55]. HS alone may not provide significant improvements to the AHI and is typically conducted as a component of comprehensive therapy [23]. In a study of female OSA patients, isolated HS consistently failed to achieve surgical success but obtained near-curative results when hyoid-mandibular suspension was conducted alongside UPPP [55].

HS functions via an artificial anteropositioning of the hyoid and thus increased anteroposterior dimensions of the airway [23]. The hyoid bone would traditionally be suspended to the lingual surface of the mandible, (**Figure 4**) though the need for an additional incision at the submental region as well as extensive dissection through the submental tissues have led to modified procedures that suspend the hyoid bone to the thyroid cartilage instead [55].

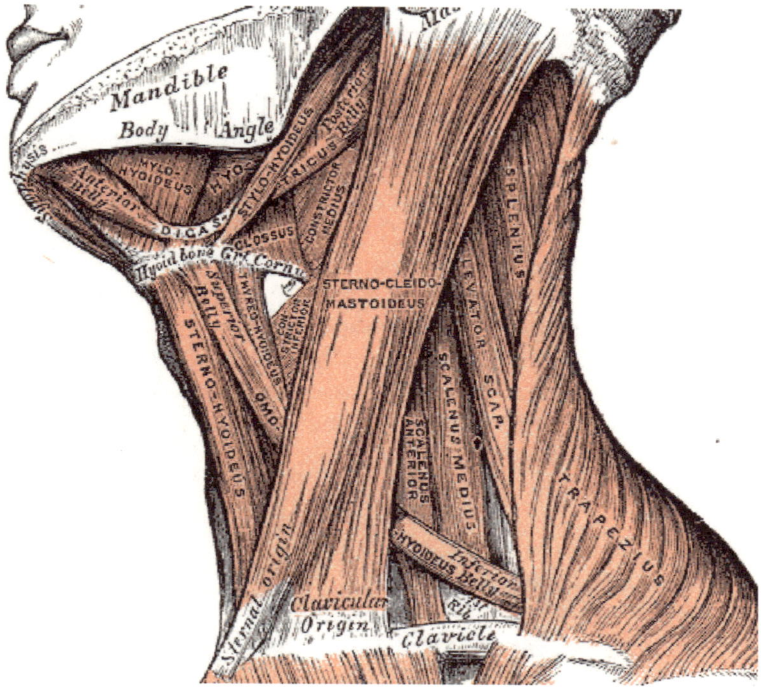

Figure 4.
Position of the hyoid bone.

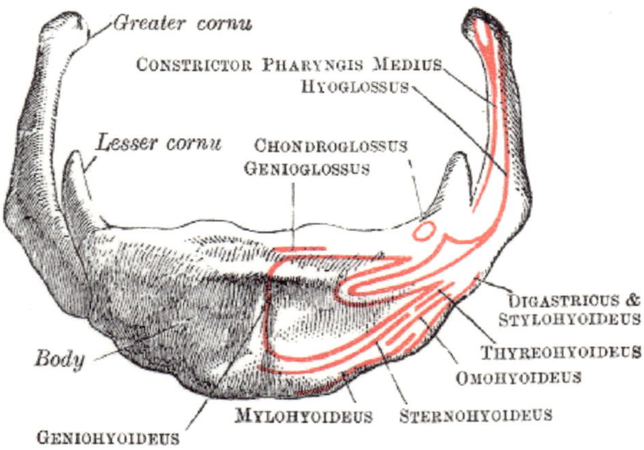

Figure 5.
The muscular and ligamentous attachment sites of the hyoid bone.

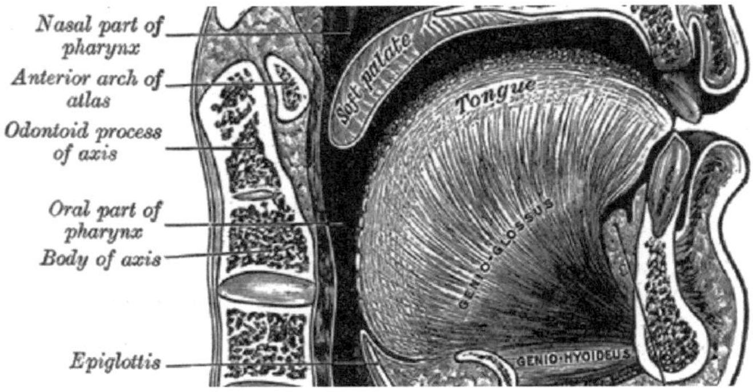

Figure 6.
Depiction of the genioglossus and its attachment site.

In both surgical variants, the hyoid bone is first approached via a direct incision. The infra-hyoid muscles are dissected from the bony surface and the stylohyoid ligaments are sectioned from the lesser cornu (**Figure 5**). In cases of hyoid suspension to the mandible, the submental region is then approached via sharp and/or blunt dissection to the lingual surface of the mandible. The digastric and mylohyoid muscles are separated laterally to avoid complete dissection from the mandible.

Two or more bony anchors are placed near the attachment site of the genioglossus (**Figure 6**). Non-resorbable sutures or wires may be wrapped around the body of the hyoid then passed through the bony anchors (in the case of hyo-mandibular suspension) or the thyroid cartilage (in the case of hyo-thyroid suspension) to advance the hyoid bone approximately 3 cm, inducing tension in its muscular attachments [23, 55]. A drain may left in place for 2 to 3 days to help reduce the risk of seroma or hematoma.

14. Genioglossus advancement

Genioglossus advancement (GA) is another surgical procedure commonly conducted in combination with HS or maxillomandibular advancement. The genioglossus muscle - and therefore, the base of the tongue – is advanced anteriorly to increase the anteroposterior diameter of the retrolingual airway [56]. While its rate of success as a standalone treatment remains at approximately 50%, this rate may increase greatly when conducted in conjunction with maxillomandibular advancement [57]. As expected, GA is not effective in treating obstructions at the palate.

GA may be performed as an anterior mandibular osteotomy to advance the genioglossus muscle without altering the external appearance of the chin. A preoperative CT scan is utilized to locate the anterior attachment site of the genioglossus at the mental spine of the mandible (**Figure 7**). An osteotomy guide – frequently made as an occlusal-based appliance to fit over the mandibular dentition - is then created to separate this site from the rest of the mandible via a rectangular bicortical osteotomy approached from the buccal side of the mandible [56].

An intraoral incision is made through the anterior mandibular buccal vestibule to reach the osteotomy site at the symphysis. The subperiosteal dissection should be extended down to the inferior border of the mandible and laterally to the regions of the bilateral canines. Once the osteotomy is conducted, the freed segment of mandibular bone is typically advanced such that the lingual cortex of the freed segment is at or anterior to the buccal cortex of the surrounding mandible. The buccal cortex and the cancellous portions of the freed segment may be trimmed away to minimize

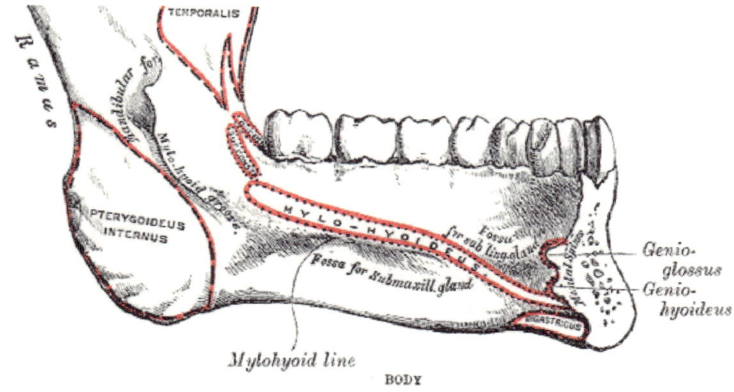

Figure 7.
Mental spine and the attachment sites of the genioglossus muscle.

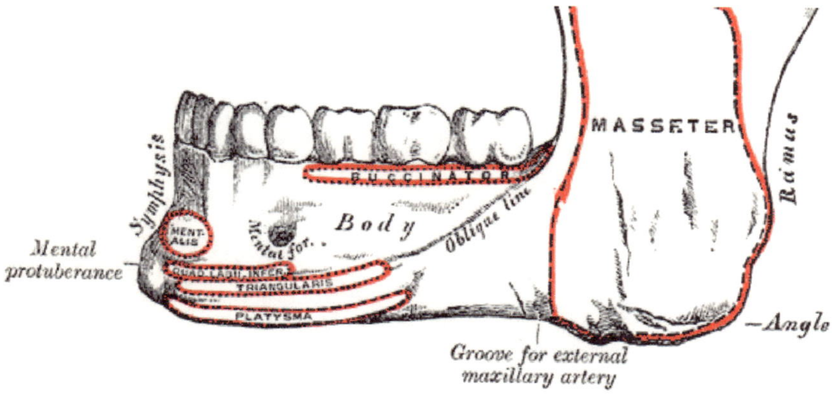

Figure 8.
Mental protuberance at the inferior aspect of the mandibular symphysis.

bony protrustion at the chin. The freed segment is fixated in place using titanium plates, which may be custom-made for convenience.

GA may also be performed as a part of cosmetically driven genioplasty in individuals with retrognathia. A large portion of the mental protuberance is advanced in addition to the segment of bone attached to the genioglossus muscle, which increases chin volume and esthetic outcome [57]. Instead of osteotomizing just the attachment site of the genioglossus, the operators would utilize an osteotomy guide that also encompasses a bulk of the mental protuberance (**Figure 8**).

15. Maxillomandibular advancement

Maxillomandibular advancement (MMA) is considered an effective surgical modality for patients affected by nasopharyngeal, retropalatal and/or retrolingual obstructions [5, 58, 59]. A recent meta-analysis suggests that MMA has greater than a 98% rate of clinical improvement, 85% rate of treatment success, and approximately 40% rate of a complete cure [59]. A potential downside of MMA treatment includes its invasiveness and applicability only in individuals who are esthetically amenable to an increasing prominence of the bimaxillary complex. Conversely, an MMA may be especially well suited for patients with hypoplastic dentofacial deformities who require such bony changes [60].

Like GA, MMA requires pre-operative planning frequently aided by CT scans. The radiographs may then be supplemented by stone models or optical scans of the patient's dentition to increase the accuracy in virtual surgical planning (VSP). Occlusal dental splints are produced which help execute the planned bony movements. MMA also frequently requires that approximately 1 year of pre-operative orthodontics be conducted to create a stable occlusion that is not only esthetic but is amenable to intermaxillary fixation (IMF).

To conduct MMA, a LeFort 1 osteotomy and a bilateral sagittal splint osteotomy (BSSO) are conducted to advance the palatal-alveolar complex and the body of the mandible, respectively (**Figure 9**). These horizontal advancements may be conducted in conjunction with a counterclockwise rotation of the maxillomandibular

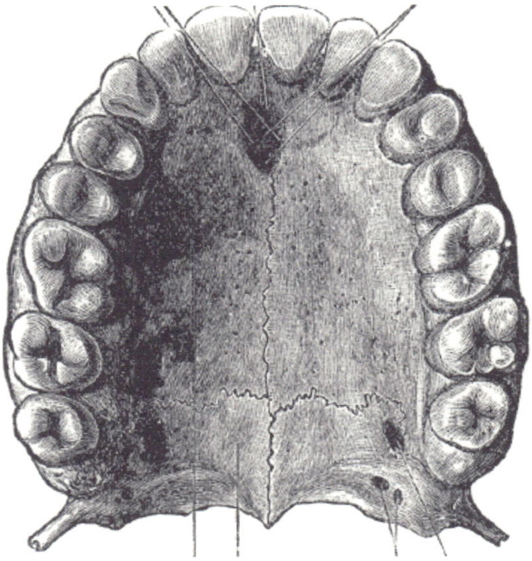

Figure 9.
The palatal-alveolar complex of the maxilla.

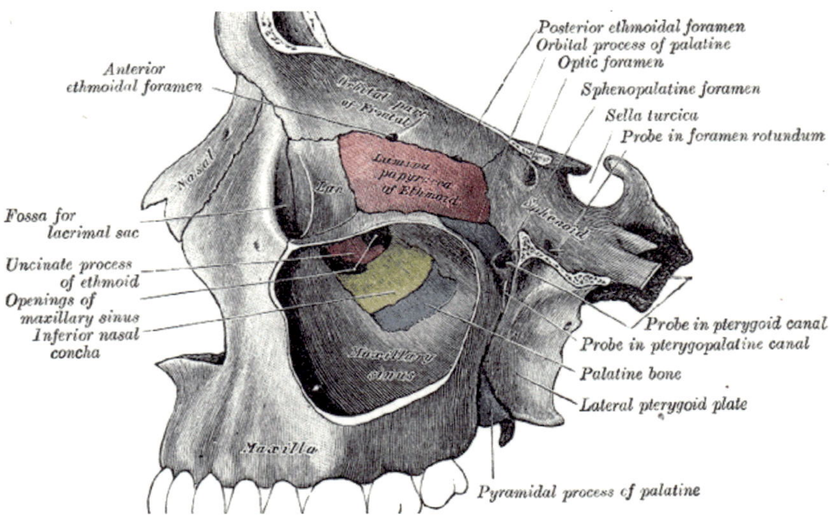

Figure 10.
The anterior, medial, lateral, and posterior walls of the maxillary sinus and their relationships to the lateral pterygoid plate.

complex (when viewed in a right lateral position) to accomplish a total advancement of the mandibular symphysis by at least 10 mm from its native position [57, 60].

Typically, the LeFort 1 osteotomy is conducted first to establish a stable upper dental position. The anterior and lateral walls of the maxilla are exposed via an incision through the maxillary buccal vestibule. A subperiosteal dissection is conducted, after which a saw osteotomy is made through the anterior and anterolateral walls of the maxillary sinuses (**Figure 10**). The osteotomies are continued posteriorly through the medial and lateral walls of the sinuses using osteotomes. The lateral pterygoid plates are also detached from the maxilla proper using a curved osteotome. The operator may elect to make a lateral approach to the pterygoid plates by gently "walking" the osteotome posteriorly along the lateral and posterior walls of the maxillary sinuses until the tip of the osteotome makes contact with a slight concavity at the pterygomaxillary junction. Gentle mallet impacts are then utilized to accomplish the detachment.

The nasal mucosae are also bluntly dissected from its attachments to the inferior and lateral walls of the nasal cavity. At this point, the posterior walls of the maxillary sinuses are the only osseous connections between the palatal-alveolar and the midface segments of the maxilla (**Figure 11**). A gentle downward pressure is applied at the anterior maxillary dentition to cause a controlled, horizontal fracture across the posterior walls of the maxillary sinuses. The soft tissue attachments to the palatal-alveolar segment are then stretched in preparation for its anterior movement.

The freed palatal-alveolar segment is then advanced approximately 10 mm via the use of preformed "intermediate" dental occlusal splints, which engages the mandibular dentition to hold the maxillary teeth approximately 10 mm anteriorly from their original positions. IMF is conducted with the splint in place (either with arch bars, pre-existing orthodontia, or intermaxillary screws) to stabilize the palatal-alveolar segment to the mandible. This allows the surgeons to trim and apply plate fixation to the palatal-alveolar segment in its new position relative to the rest of the maxilla.

The BSSO is performed next, although some providers may elect to perform the BSSO first followed by the LeFort 1 osteotomy. IMF is released and incisions are made through the bilateral buccal vestibules of the mandible to reveal the lateral

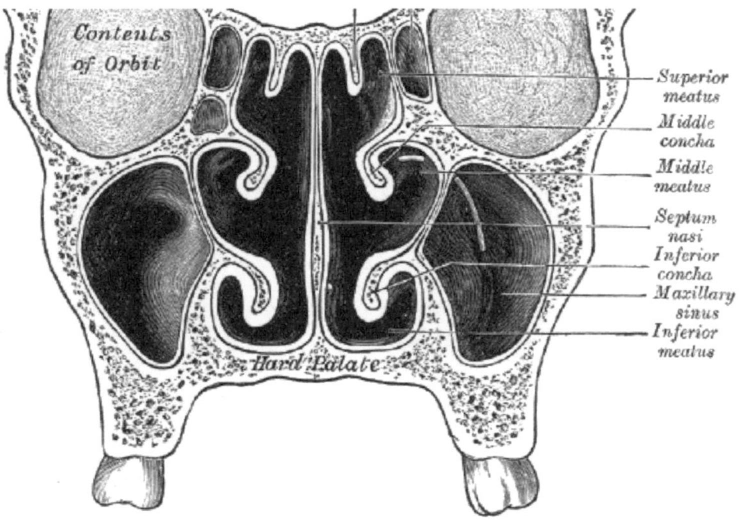

Figure 11.
A coronal section demonstrating the darkened, intact posterior walls of the maxillary sinuses.

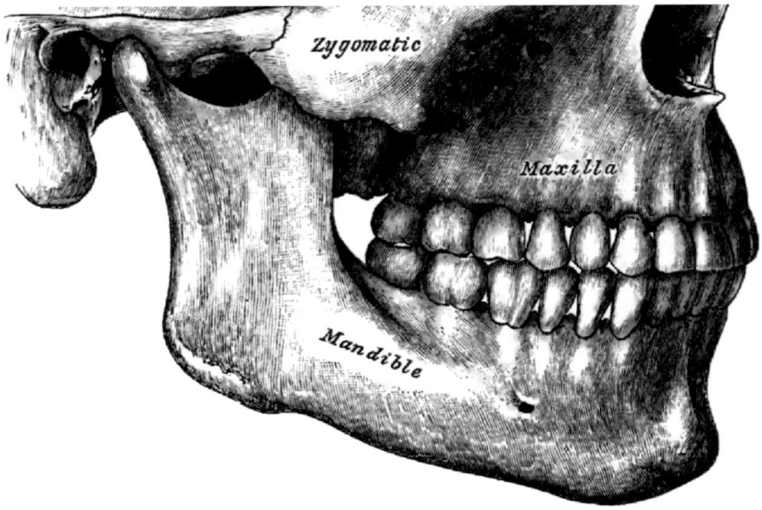

Figure 12.
The maxillomandibular complex. BSSO are conducted through the superolateral cortex of the mandibular body just medial to the ramus and just lateral to the posterior dention.

cortex of the mandibular body as well as the antero-medial surfaces of the ramus. A monocortical saw osteotomy is then started from a point just superior to the lingula and continued downwards along the superolateral cortex of the mandibular body until it reaches the cortex just lateral to the first molar (**Figure 12**). The positioning of this osteotomy reduces the risk of injury to the inferior alveolar neurovascular bundle at its entrance and through its canal. Gentle osteotome pressure is applied through the osteotomies to propagate controlled fractures at the posterior wall of each ramus and the inferior wall of each mandibular body.

Once the body of the mandible is freed from its bilateral ramus-condyle segments, preformed "final' dental occlusal splint may be used to advance the mandibular body segment. The splint engages the now-stable maxillary dentition to hold the mandibular teeth approximately 10 mm anteriorly from their original positions. IMF is again conducted with the new splint in place. The mandibular segment may be fixated in its new position (using orthopedic plates) relative to the bilateral ramus-condyle segments. After releasing the IMF and confirming correct occlusion, the patient should be re-placed in IMF for approximately two weeks followed by four additional weeks of non-chew diet.

The BSSO should be conducted first in cases where the pre-operative CT scans were taken without the condylar heads seated in the temporal fossa. The condyles may be seated after a proper mandibular advancement, and the new mandibular dental occlusion may then be used as the reference against which the palatal-alveolar segment is advanced.

16. Hypoglossal nerve stimulator

The hypoglossal nerve stimulator (HGNS) is a newly developed device that activates the hypoglossal nerve upon detection of an apneic episode. It includes a sensing and a stimulating electrode, which detects then mitigates apnea, respectively. HGNS is particularly effective in individuals with non-concentric, antero-posterior collapse of the retrolingual airway on DISE. It demonstrated a median AHI improvement of 68% in individuals with BMIs under 32 kg/m^2 [61]. After implantation, the HGNS impulses may be adjusted according to the patient's post-operative AHI and/or RDI

DOI: http://dx.doi.org/10.5772/intechopen.95072

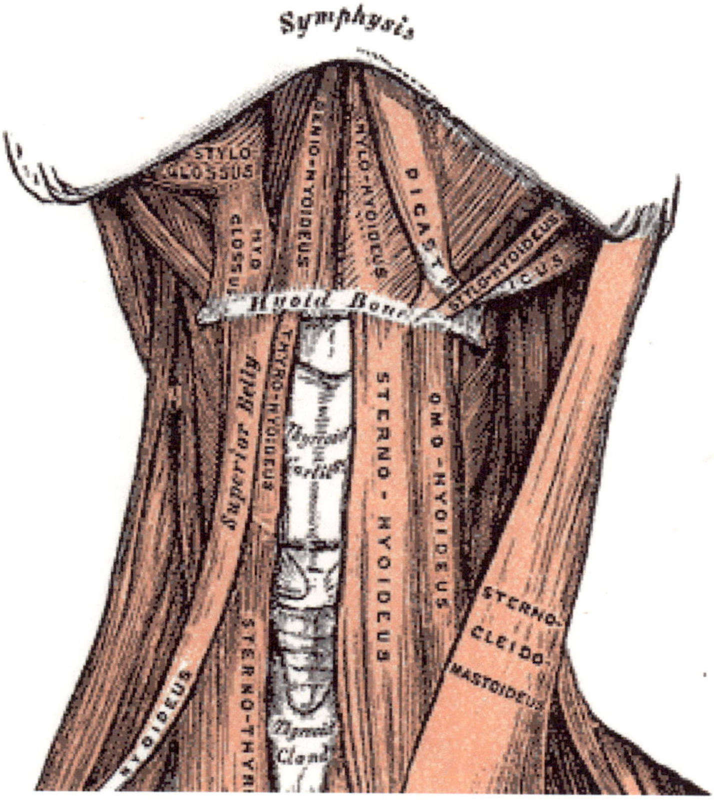

Figure 13.
Main anatomic landmarks for HGNS surgery including the hyoid bone and the digastric muscles.

values. Higher impulse charges may be avoided in sensitive individuals who are awakened by a sudden activation of the hypoglossal nerve.

To place the HGNS, a submandibular incision is first made approximately 2 cm below the inferior border of the mandible to avoid the marginal mandibular branch of the facial nerve. The site is dissected until the hyoid bone is appreciated, followed by a slight lateral extension to identify the posterior and anterior bellies of the digastric muscle (**Figure 13**). The digastric tendon is identified and isolated from the surrounding soft tissues using retractors. The hypoglossal nerve is found in the space medial to the digastric muscle just lateral to the hyoid bone. It is close to the Ranine vein which lies immediately posterior.

The Ranine vein may be ligated and the hypoglossal nerve further dissected anteriorly from the surrounding tissues to locate its "inclusion" and "exclusion" branches. The inclusion branches are those that protrude the tongue and the exclusion branches are those that retrude it. The two branches may be distinguished with a stimulator, and the HGNS stimulating electrode is cuffed to the primary inclusion branch. The electrode itself should be secured to the digastric tendon using nonresorbable sutures to prevent dislocation from the nerve.

The upper chest incision is then made approximately 4 cm below the mid-clavicle down to the pectoralis fascia, which is left intact. A supra-fascial dissection is made to create a small cavity for the pulse generator. A lateral chest incision is also needed about 2 cm below and 5 cm laterally from the nipple for the implantation of the sensing lead. The approach is continued through the serratus anterior and external intercostal muscles to secure the sensing electrode in a plane between the external and internal intercostal muscles (**Figure 14**). The internal intercostal muscles must be left intact to avoid pneumothorax.

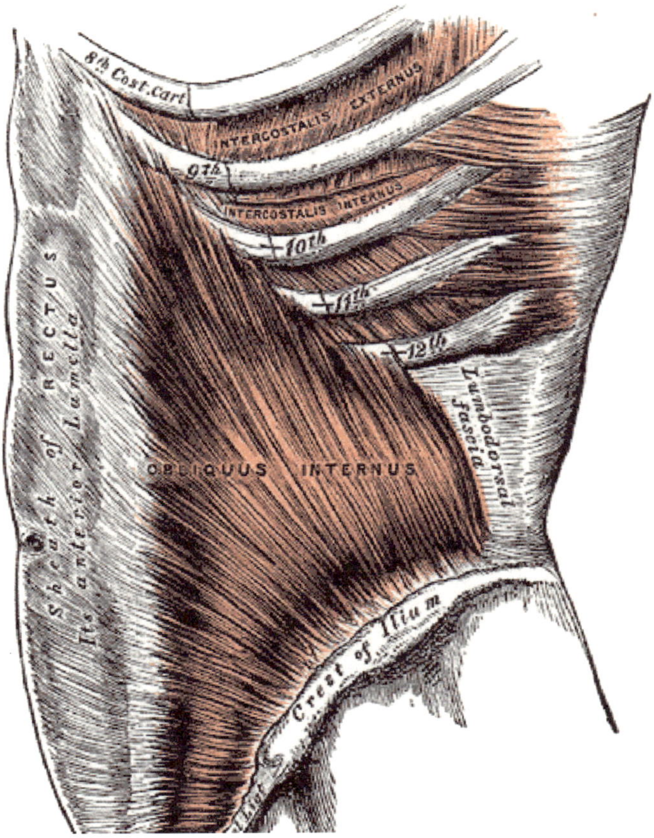

Figure 14.
The external and internal intercostal muscles.

The sensing electrode wires are tunneled subcutaneously from the lateral chest site to the pulse generator at the upper chest site. Similarly, the stimulating electrode wires are also tunneled in a sub-platysmal plate from the neck site to the pulse generator. The pulse generator is sutured in place at the upper chest pocket and connected to the respective electrode wires. The generator's power supply should be replaced approximately every ten years.

16.1 Tracheostomy

Tracheostomy is perhaps the oldest and the most definitive intervention for OSA. An incision is made through the anterior neck to insert a semi-permanent airway, bypassing both the naso- and oropharynx. Though it is typically performed to establish an emergency airway and/or to create a long-term ventilation port, it may be performed in cases of severe obstructive sleep apnea that is otherwise refractory to other treatment modalities. Tracheostomy is considered a treatment of last resort owing to its invasive nature and a relatively high rate of complications such as hemorrhage, tracheal stenosis, tracheoesophageal or tracheocutaneous fistula, and bronchospasm regardless of the approach taken [62, 63]. A recent systematic review indicated that percutaneous dilatational tracheostomy carries an overall mortality rate of approximately 1 in 600 [64]. It also requires dedicated maintenance including frequent suctioning and regular replacement of its parts.

Elective tracheostomy for OSA should be conducted in a sterile fashion in the operating room. A horizontal incision is made approximately 2 cm superior to the

DOI: http://dx.doi.org/10.5772/intechopen.95072

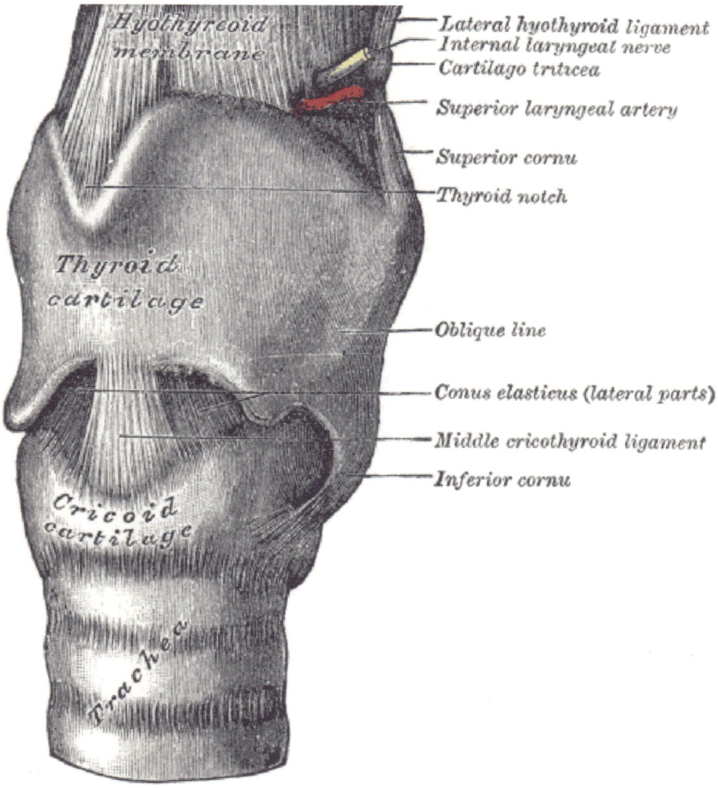

Figure 15.
The anatomy of the thyroid, cricoid, and tracheal cartilages.

suprasternal notch then dissected through the subcutaneous and platysmal layers. The subsequent fascia and strap muscles are divided along a vertical line until the thyroid gland or the pretracheal fascia are encountered. Any thyroid tissues encountered may be retracted superiorly, and the pretracheal fascia bluntedly dissected away from the airway.

At this point, the patient's FiO2 should be lowered and the endotracheal tube advanced further to avoid the risk of fire and cuff puncture, respectively. A horizontal incision is first made between the tracheal rings (**Figure 15**). This is connected to a vertical, downward incision through the tracheal ring just below from each end of the horizontal incision to raise a Bjork flap. Resorbable sutures are passed under the cartilagenous ring to fixate the flap to the overlying skin. An appropriately sized tracheostomy tube is inserted atraumatically then stabilized to the neck using a trap. The endotracheal tube may be removed, and the tracheostomy tube cuff inflated.

17. Pediatric OSA

In general, both the prevalence and treatment threshold for OSA in children is lower [65]. Children with AHI greater than 5 should undergo treatment to help normalize breathing. For patients with AHI ranging from 1 to 5, treatment should be considered if OSA-related comorbidities such as obesity, hyperactive behaviors, lymphoid hyperplasia, enuresis, and/or increased inflammatory markers are present [65, 66]. Non-invasive measures like weight loss and avoidance of irritants like tobacco smoking are universally helpful [65].

Most literature indicate an OSA incidence of 1 to 4% [67]. This occurrence peaks between the ages of 2 to 8, which roughly coincides with the peak instances of lymphoid hyperplasia. Traditional treatment therefore consists of tonsillectomy with or without adenoidectomy. However, the success rate may range as low as 27% even though delaying correction of disordered breathing can lead to gnathic or craniofacial anomalies [66]. While removal of tonsillar or adenoidal tissues can be conducted at any age, other surgical interventions may incur a greater rate of complications (in non-syndromic patients) if conducted prior to age 3 or in individuals weighing less than 15 kg [65, 68].

Alternative surgical modalities include septoplasty and UPPP. Osseous surgeries should be reserved for those with craniofacial deficits as extensive osteotomies frequently disrupt the rate and pattern of skeletal growth. Maxillary and/or mandibular distraction may be employed early to utilize the rapid healing potential in children with severe micrognathia [65].

Unlike in adults, CPAP should be reserved for moderate or severe cases of pediatric OSA that cannot be treated surgically [69]. CPAP compliance rate is even lower in children, and a lack of appropriate pediatric CPAP appliances as well as long sleeping hours exacerbate this issue [70]. CPAP can also trigger nasal symptoms such as congestion, epistaxis, and midface retrusion [65]. Patients who cannot tolerate or are refractory to surgery and CPAP should undergo treatment via tracheostomy [69].

18. Surveillance

Post-intervention polysomnography or DISE may be conducted at least 3 months after therapy to reduce confounding effects of post-operative edema. STOP-BANG, Epworth, and/or Berlin questionnaires should also be utilized to ensure improvements in the patient's quality of life.

The Stanford Protocol is a predictable and effective protocol outlining the proper elevation of care in cases of OSA relapse [71]. Surgical management of OSA should begin with the phase 1 treatments consisting of septoplasty, UPPP, then GA. Phase 2 treatment is MMA and may be conducted in case of relapse after phase 1. While phase 2 treatment appears sufficient for most patients, a recent update to the Protocol showed that HGNS could be conducted in cases of phase 2 treatment failure [72]. MMA may prevent lateral pharyngeal wall components of airway collapse, thereby increasing the efficacy of HGNS which best addresses antero-posterior obstructions.

19. Conclusions

Obstructive sleep apnea is a complex disease of numerous significant ramifications which require careful diagnosis and management. As with many chronic conditions, OSA should be first approached via conservative treatment which often remains equally or more effective as their invasive counterparts. Once the reversible conservative modalities are exhausted, the more invasive therapies should be approached with caution. Modern interventional protocols like the Stanford Protocol may provide guidance based on the successes of large volume surgical cohorts.

Acknowledgements

The anatomic figures in this chapter (**Figures 1** through **13**) have been obtained from the work of Drs. Henry Gray and Henry Vandyke Carter within the public domain of the United States of America.

Conflict of interest

The authors declare no conflicts of interest.

Author details

Ho-Hyun (Brian) Sun[1]* and Sally Sun[2]

1 University of California, San Francisco – Highland Hospital, Kaiser Permanente Oakland Medical Center, Western University of Health Sciences, College of Dental Medicine, Dublin, California, USA

2 University of the Pacific, Thomas J. Long School of Pharmacy, Kaiser Permanente Dublin Medical Offices and Cancer Center, Dublin, California, USA

*Address all correspondence to: hsun@westernu.edu

References

[1] Senaratna C V, Perret JL, Lodge CJ, Lowe AJ, Campbell BE, Matheson MC, et al. Prevalence of obstructive sleep apnea in the general population : A systematic review. Sleep Medicine Reviews. 2020;34(2017):70-81.

[2] Franklin KA, Lindberg E. Obstructive sleep apnea is a common disorder in the population-A review on the epidemiology of sleep apnea. Vol. 7, Journal of Thoracic Disease. 2015. p. 1311-22.

[3] Schwab RJ, Kim C, Bagchi S, Keenan BT, Comyn FL, Wang S, et al. Understanding the anatomic basis for obstructive sleep apnea syndrome in adolescents. American Journal of Respiratory and Critical Care Medicine. 2015;191(11):1295-309.

[4] Caporale M, Palmeri R, Corallo F, Muscarà N, Romeo L, Bramanti A, et al. Cognitive impairment in obstructive sleep apnea syndrome: a descriptive review. Sleep and Breathing. 2020;

[5] Pirklbauer K, Russmueller G, Stiebellehner L, Nell C, Sinko K, Millesi G, et al. Maxillomandibular advancement for treatment of obstructive sleep apnea syndrome: A systematic review. Journal of Oral and Maxillofacial Surgery. 2011;69(6):e165-76.

[6] De Miguel-Díez J, Villa-Asensi JR, Álvarez-Sala JL. Prevalence of sleep-disordered breathing in children with down syndrome: Polygraphic findings in 108 children. Sleep. 2003;26(8):1006-9.

[7] Bray GA. What's in a Name? Mr. Dickens' "Pickwickian" Fat Boy Syndrome. Obesity Research. 1994;2(4):380-3.

[8] Sullivan C, Berthon-Jones M, Issa F, Eves L. Reversal of Obstructive Sleep Apnoea by Continuous Positive Airway Pressure Applied Through the Nares. The Lancet. 1981;317(8225):862-5.

[9] Goyal A, Pakhare AP, Bhatt GC, Choudhary B, Patil R. Association of pediatric obstructive sleep apnea with poor academic performance: A school-based study from India. Lung India : official organ of Indian Chest Society. 2018;35(2):132-6.

[10] McNicholas WT. Diagnosis of obstructive sleep apnea in adults. Proceedings of the American Thoracic Society. 2008 Feb;5(2):154-60.

[11] Saboisky JP, Butler JE, Gandevia SC, Eckert DJ. Functional role of neural injury in obstructive sleep apnea. Frontiers in Neurology. 2012;JUN(June):1-12.

[12] Krysta K, Bratek A, Zawada K, Stepańczak R. Cognitive deficits in adults with obstructive sleep apnea compared to children and adolescents. Journal of Neural Transmission. 2017;124:187-201.

[13] Foldvary-Schaefer NR, Waters TE. Sleep-Disordered Breathing. CONTINUUM: Lifelong Learning in Neurology. 2017;23(4).

[14] Dehlink E, Tan H-L. Update on paediatric obstructive sleep apnoea. Journal of thoracic disease. 2016 Feb;8(2):224-35.

[15] Sleep-Related Breathing Disorders in Adults: Recommendations for Syndrome Definition and Measurement Techniques in Clinical Research. Sleep. 1999 Aug 1;22(5):667-89.

[16] Kapur VK, Auckley DH, Chowdhuri S, Kuhlmann DC, Mehra R, Ramar K, et al. Clinical Practice Guideline for Diagnostic Testing for Adult Obstructive Sleep Apnea. Journal of Clinical Sleep Medicine. 2017;1313(3):479-504.

[17] Kotecha B, De Vito A. Drug induced sleep endoscopy: Its role in evaluation of the upper airway obstruction and patient selection for surgical and nonsurgical treatment. Journal of Thoracic Disease. 2018;10(1):S40-7.

[18] Johns MW. A new method for measuring daytime sleepiness: The Epworth sleepiness scale. Sleep. 1991;14(6):540-5.

[19] Netzer NC, Stoohs RA, Netzer CM, Clark K, Strohl KP. Using the Berlin Questionnaire To Identify Patients at Risk for the Sleep Apnea Syndrome. Annals of Internal Medicine. 1999 Oct 5;131(7):485-91.

[20] Vasu TS, Doghramji K, Cavallazzi R, Grewal R, Hirani A, Leiby B, et al. Obstructive Sleep Apnea Syndrome and Postoperative Complications: Clinical Use of the STOP-BANG Questionnaire. Archives of Otolaryngology–Head & Neck Surgery. 2010 Oct 18;136(10):1020-4.

[21] Chiu HY, Chen PY, Chuang LP, Chen NH, Tu YK, Hsieh YJ, et al. Diagnostic accuracy of the Berlin questionnaire, STOP-BANG, STOP, and Epworth sleepiness scale in detecting obstructive sleep apnea: A bivariate meta-analysis. Sleep Medicine Reviews. 2017;36(2017):57-70.

[22] Amra B, Javani M, Soltaninejad F, Penzel T, Fietze I, Schoebel C, et al. Comparison of Berlin Questionnaire, STOP-Bang, and Epworth Sleepiness Scale for Diagnosing Obstructive Sleep Apnea in Persian Patients. International journal of preventive medicine. 2018 Mar 9;9:28.

[23] Stuck BA, Neff W, Hörmann K, Verse T, Bran G, Baisch A, et al. Anatomic changes after hyoid suspension for obstructive sleep apnea: An MRI study. Otolaryngology - Head and Neck Surgery. 2005;133(3):397-402.

[24] Qaseem A, Holty J-EC, Owens DK, Dallas P, Starkey M, Shekelle P. Management of Obstructive Sleep Apnea in Adults: A Clinical Practice Guideline From the American College of Physicians. Annals of Internal Medicine. 2013 Oct 1;159(7):471-83.

[25] Iftikhar IH, Kline CE, Youngstedt SD. Effects of exercise training on sleep apnea: A meta-analysis. Lung. 2014;192(1):175-84.

[26] Azagra-Calero E, Espinar-Escalona E, Barrera-Mora JM, Llamas-Carreras JM, Solano-Reina E. Obstructive sleep apnea syndrome (OSAS). Review of the literature. Medicina Oral, Patologia Oral y Cirugia Bucal. 2012;17(6).

[27] Neill AMK, Angus SM, Sajkov D, McEvoy RD. Effects of sleep posture on upper airway stability in patients with obstructive sleep apnea. American Journal of Respiratory and Critical Care Medicine. 1997;155(1):199-204.

[28] Nakano H, Ikeda T, Hayashi M, Ohshima E, Onizuka A. Effects of body position on snoring in apneic and nonapneic snorers. Sleep. 2003;26(2):169-72.

[29] Ward CP, York KM, McCoy JG. Risk of obstructive sleep apnea lower in double reed wind musicians. Journal of Clinical Sleep Medicine. 2012;8(3):251-5.

[30] BUCKS RS, OLAITHE M, EASTWOOD P. Neurocognitive function in obstructive sleep apnoea: A meta-review. Respirology. 2013 Jan 1;18(1):61-70.

[31] Jackson ML, McEvoy RD, Banks S, Barnes M. Neurobehavioral impairment and CPAP treatment response in mild-moderate obstructive sleep apnea. Journal of Clinical Sleep Medicine. 2018;14(1):47-56.

[32] Drager LF, Togeiro SM, Polotsky VY, Lorenzi-Filho G. Obstructive sleep apnea: A cardiometabolic risk in obesity and the metabolic syndrome. Journal of the American College of Cardiology. 2013;62(7):569-76.

[33] Zozula R, Rosen R. Compliance with continuous positive airway pressure therapy: assessing and improving treatment outcomes. Current opinion in pulmonary medicine. 2001 Nov;7(6):391-8.

[34] Morgenthaler TI, Aurora RN, Brown T, Zak R, Alessi C, Boehlecke B, et al. Practice parameters for the use of autotitrating continuous positive airway pressure devices for titrating pressures and treating adult patients with obstructive sleep apnea syndrome: An update for 2007 - An American Academy of Sleep Medicine Report. Sleep. 2008;31(1):141-7.

[35] Ramar K, Dort LC, Katz SG, Lettieri CJ, Harrod CG, Thomas SM, et al. Clinical Practice Guideline for the Treatment of Obstructive Sleep Apnea and Snoring with Oral Appliance Therapy: An Update for 2015. Journal of clinical sleep medicine : JCSM : official publication of the American Academy of Sleep Medicine. 2015 Jul 15;11(7):773-827.

[36] Pantin CC, Hillman DR, Tennant M. Dental side effects of an oral device to treat snoring and obstructive sleep apnea. Sleep. 1999;22(2):237-40.

[37] Gaisl T, Haile SR, Thiel S, Osswald M, Kohler M. Efficacy of pharmacotherapy for OSA in adults: A systematic review and network meta-analysis. Sleep Medicine Reviews. 2019;46(2019):74-86.

[38] Fenik P, Veasey SC. Pharmacological characterization of serotonergic receptor activity in the hypoglossal nucleus. American journal of respiratory and critical care medicine. 2003;167(4):563-9.

[39] Carley DW, Olopade C, Ruigt GS, Radulovacki M. Efficacy of mirtazapine in obstructive sleep apnea syndrome. Sleep. 2007;30(1):35-41.

[40] Kraiczi H, Hedner J, Dahlöf P, Ejnell H, Carlson J. Effect of serotonin uptake inhibition on breathing during sleep and daytime symptoms in obstructive sleep apnea. Sleep. 1999;22(1):61-7.

[41] Carley DW, Radulovacki M. Role of Peripheral Serotonin in the Regulation of Central Sleep Apneas in Rats. Chest. 1999;115(5):1397-401.

[42] Sukys-Claudino L, Moraes W, Guilleminault C, Tufik S, Poyares D. Beneficial effect of donepezil on obstructive sleep apnea: A double-blind, placebo-controlled clinical trial. Sleep Medicine. 2012;13(3):290-6.

[43] Hein H, Behnke G, Jörres RA, Magnussen H. The therapeutic effect of theophylline in mild obstructive sleep Apnea/Hypopnea syndrome: results of repeated measurements with portable recording devices at home. European journal of medical research. 2000 Sep;5(9):391-9.

[44] Prasad B, Radulovacki M, Olopade C, Herdegen JJ, Logan T, Carley DW. Prospective trial of efficacy and safety of ondansetron and fluoxetine in patients with obstructive sleep apnea syndrome. Sleep. 2010;33(7):982-9.

[45] Carley DW, Prasad B, Reid KJ, Malkani R, Attarian H, Abbott SM, et al. Pharmacotherapy of apnea by cannabimimetic enhancement, the PACE clinical trial: Effects of dronabinol in obstructive sleep apnea. Sleep. 2018;41(1).

[46] Weaver EM, Maynard C, Yueh B. Survival of Veterans With Sleep Apnea: Continuous Positive Airway Pressure Versus Surgery. Otolaryngology–Head

and Neck Surgery. 2004 Jun 1;130(6):659-65.

[47] Lin H-C, Friedman M, Chang H-W, Gurpinar B. The Efficacy of Multilevel Surgery of the Upper Airway in Adults With Obstructive Sleep Apnea/Hypopnea Syndrome. The Laryngoscope. 2008 May 1;118(5):902-8.

[48] Stuck BA, Leitzbach S, Maurer JT. Effects of continuous positive airway pressure on apnea–hypopnea index in obstructive sleep apnea based on long-term compliance. Sleep and Breathing. 2012;16(2):467-71.

[49] Venekamp RP, Hearne BJ, Chandrasekharan D, Blackshaw H, Lim J, Schilder AG. Tonsillectomy or adenotonsillectomy versus non-surgical management for obstructive sleep-disordered breathing in children (Review) SUMMARY OF FINDINGS FOR THE MAIN COMPARISON. The Cochrane Library. 2015;(10):CD011165.

[50] Pinder DK, Wilson H, Hilton MP. Dissection versus diathermy for tonsillectomy. Cochrane Database of Systematic Reviews. 2011;

[51] Windfuhr JP, Chen YS, Remmert S. Hemorrhage following tonsillectomy and adenoidectomy in 15,218 patients. Otolaryngology–Head and Neck Surgery. 2005 Feb 1;132(2):281-6.

[52] Li H-Y, Wang P-C, Chen Y-P, Lee L-A, Fang T-J, Lin H-C. Critical Appraisal and Meta-Analysis of Nasal Surgery for Obstructive Sleep Apnea. American Journal of Rhinology & Allergy. 2011 Jan 1;25(1):45-9.

[53] Mickelson SA. Nasal Surgery for Obstructive Sleep Apnea Syndrome. Otolaryngologic Clinics of North America. 2016;49(6):1373-81.

[54] Yousuf A, Beigh Z, Khursheed RS, Jallu AS, Pampoori RA. Clinical predictors for successful uvulopalatopharyngoplasty in the management of obstructive sleep apnea. International journal of otolaryngology. 2013/09/19. 2013;2013:290265.

[55] Mickelson SA. Hyoid advancement to the mandible (hyo-mandibular advancement). Operative Techniques in Otolaryngology - Head and Neck Surgery. 2012;23(1):56-9.

[56] Cheng A. Genioglossus and Genioplasty Advancement. Atlas of the Oral and Maxillofacial Surgery Clinics of North America. 2019;27(1):23-8.

[57] Liao YF, Chiu YT, Lin CH, Chen YA, Chen NH, Chen YR. Modified maxillomandibular advancement for obstructive sleep apnoea: Towards a better outcome for Asians. International Journal of Oral and Maxillofacial Surgery. 2015;44(2):189-94.

[58] PRINSELL JR. Maxillomandibular advancement surgery for obstructive sleep apnea syndrome. The Journal of the American Dental Association. 2002 Nov 1;133(11):1489-97.

[59] Zaghi S, Holty JEC, Certal V, Abdullatif J, Guilleminault C, Powell NB, et al. Maxillomandibular advancement for treatment of obstructive sleep apnea ameta-analysis. JAMA Otolaryngology - Head and Neck Surgery. 2016;142(1):58-66.

[60] Liu SYC, Awad M, Riley RW. Maxillomandibular Advancement: Contemporary Approach at Stanford. Atlas of the Oral and Maxillofacial Surgery Clinics of North America. 2019;27(1):29-36.

[61] Strollo PJ, Soose RJ, Maurer JT, De Vries N, Cornelius J, Froymovich O, et al. Upper-airway stimulation for obstructive sleep apnea. New England Journal of Medicine. 2014;370(2):139-49.

[62] Ferlito A, Rinaldo A, Shaha AR, Bradley PJ. Percutaneous Tracheotomy. Acta Oto-Laryngologica. 2003 Sep 1;123(9):1008-12.

[63] Klemm E, Nowak AK. Tracheotomy-related deaths-a systematic review. Deutsches Arzteblatt International. 2017;114(16).

[64] Simon M, Metschke M, Braune SA, Püschel K, Kluge S. Death after percutaneous dilatational tracheostomy: A systematic review and analysis of risk factors. Critical Care. 2013;17(5).

[65] Ahn YM. Treatment of obstructive sleep apnea in children. Korean Journal of Pediatrics. 2010;53(10):872-9.

[66] Guilleminault C, Lee JH, Chan A. Pediatric Obstructive Sleep Apnea Syndrome. Archives of Pediatrics & Adolescent Medicine. 2005 Aug 1;159(8):775-85.

[67] Marcus CL, Chapman D, Ward SD, McColley SA, Herrerias CT, Stillwell PC, et al. Clinical practice guideline: Diagnosis and management of childhood obstructive sleep apnea syndrome. Pediatrics. 2002;109(4):704-12.

[68] Katz ES, D'Ambrosio CM. Pathophysiology of pediatric obstructive sleep apnea. Proceedings of the American Thoracic Society. 2008;5(2):253-62.

[69] Powell S, Kubba H, O'Brien C, Tremlett M. Paediatric obstructive sleep apnoea. BMJ (Online). 2010;340(7754):1018-23.

[70] Marcus CL, Rosen G, Davidson Ward SL, Halbower AC, Sterni L, Lutz J, et al. Adherence to and effectiveness of positive airway pressure therapy in children with obstructive sleep apnea. Pediatrics. 2006;117(3).

[71] Holty JEC, Guilleminault C. Maxillomandibular advancement for the treatment of obstructive sleep apnea: A systematic review and meta-analysis. Sleep Medicine Reviews. 2010;14(5):287-97.

[72] Liu SY, Riley RW. Continuing the Original Stanford Sleep Surgery Protocol From Upper Airway Reconstruction to Upper Airway Stimulation: Our First Successful Case. Journal of Oral and Maxillofacial Surgery. 2017;75(7):1514-8.

Section 4

Novel Considerations in Head and Neck Surgery

Chapter 8

Strategies for the Practice of Otolaryngology and Head and Neck Surgery during COVID-19 Pandemic

Juan Manuel Maza-Solano, Antonio Jiménez-Luna, Pablo Parente-Arias, Juan Carlos Amor-Dorado, Christian Calvo-Henriquez and Guillermo Plaza-Mayor

Abstract

The appearance of a new coronavirus disease called COVID-19 at the end of 2019 and its pandemic expansion in the world has changed the usual practice of medicine, and has had great impact in the field of Otorhinolaryngology and Head and Neck Surgery (OHNS). The aim of this document is to review the available evidence and propose strategies and recommendations for the medical-surgical practice of OHNS, which allow establishing the usual activity, adapting the safety and efficacy standards to the current pandemic situation. Therefore, it is required to identify and classify patients according to criteria of infectious-immunological status, and to establish recommendations for protection in consultations, hospitalization and the operating room, which avoid the transmission of the disease to other users and healthcare personnel, in the specific context of the development of our specialty. This document is the result of the collaboration of all the scientific commissions of Spanish OHNS society and therefore might help other OHNS to develop their work during COVID-19 pandemic.

Keywords: COVID-19, surgery, otolaryngology, practice, office

1. Introduction

The SARS CoV-2 disease (COVID-19) has caused millions of deaths worldwide since the pandemic status was declared by the World Health Organization (WHO) in March 2020 [1]. The SARS-CoV-2 virus, whose origin is suspected to be associated with bats or peanuts [2], is a single-stranded RNA-virus of the Coronaviridae family, closely related to the viruses responsible for severe acute respiratory syndrome (SARS) and Middle East respiratory syndrome (MERS). The main routes of entry of the virus are the mucosae of the oral and nasal cavities. Transmission occurs through direct contact from contaminated hands, fomites, or through airborne aerosols expelled when coughing, sneezing, screaming, singing, speaking, or breathing [3, 4]. The incubation period varies between 2 and 14 days (5.7 days on average) [5], after which the patient may be asymptomatic [6] or may manifest symptoms including fever, dry cough, dyspnea, myalgia, fatigue, headache, diarrhea, general malaise, anosmia, hyposmia and dysgeusia. The disease course is usually limited, although it can progress to bilateral pneumonia, respiratory distress, and death. The fatality rate of the disease is estimated to be 0.68% [7] but highly dependent on age and concurrent risk factors [8].

One of the greatest difficulties in controlling the disease is the possibility of transmission of the etiological agent by asymptomatic and presymptomatic patients. Still, the transmissibility of COVID-19 likely correlates with the onset of symptoms, with the risk lower and the lowest in presymptomatic and asymptomatic patients, respectively [9].

Health workers represent a significant percentage of the general population infected [10]. Among physicians, otorhinolaryngologists and head and neck surgeons may be at an even greater risk as a result of their frequent proximity to the upper airway and the generation of bioaerosols in their procedures [11, 12]. In fact, the infection rate of Spanish otorhinolaryngologists rose to 16.5% during the first two waves [13]. As is such, the objective of this chapter is to provide a consensus on the management of head and neck patients during the COVID-19 era based on a compilation of the best evidence adapted to the risk of transmission [14, 15].

2. Diagnosis and screening of COVID-19 patients

2.1 Diagnosis

1. Presence of the virus

   a. Detection of viral RNA: Using reverse transcriptase and polymerase chain reaction (RT-PCR), the presence of specific genes of the SARS-CoV-2 virus is determined in samples from different areas of the airway. In patients with asymptomatic, presymptomatic, or mild forms of presentation, positive RT-PCR does not necessarily confirm nor disprove transmissiblity. RT qPCR, a subtype of RT-PCR, provides a quantitative estimate by means of fluorescence that increases proportionally to the amount of nucleic acid amplified. This test reports the viral load present in the sample by detecting a specified threshold in a certain number of cycles (Ct or cycle threshold) in RT-PCR [16, 17].

   b. Presence of virus antigens (S, M and E antigens) in airway secretions: While accessible, this test shows a high number of false negatives depending on the patient's current stage of the disease. This rapid viral antigen detection test may still be effective in symptomatic patients in the outpatient setting or in large population screenings. It is highly sensitive in patients with symptoms of disease and with less than 5 days of disease progression. Despite this high sensitivity, a negative test does not confirm an absence of disease especially if suspicious symptoms are present, at which point an RT-PCR test is recommended [18].

2. Detection of antibodies in serum: In severe COVID-19 patients at least 7 days since the onset of symptoms, the detection of IgM antibodies has been considered a sign of the patient's immune response [19]. Up to 20% of patients with mild forms of COVID-19 do not produce detectoble serum antibodies [17, 20]. Production of the longer-lasting IgG antibodies begin approximately 14 days after the onset of symptoms and may incur long-term immunity to disease. IgM or IgG antibodies may have some value in the diagnosis of patients with

negative RT-PCR results but with continued COVID-19 symptoms since the seroconversion of specific IgM and IgG antibodies have been detected as early as the 4th day after the onset of symptoms

The antibody study can be performed by:

a. Rapid antibody detection tests, which are based on immunochromatography (lateral flow technique) and have become popular as "rapid tests" for antibody detection [20]. The Spanish Society of Immunology recommends its use for epidemiological studies in high risk groups [21].

b. Laboratory tests to measure the level of antibodies, which use enzyme-linked immunosorbent assay (ELISA) or chemiluminescence assay (CLIA). They are quantitative tests (specifically, CLIA has a sensitivity of 1 pg./ml in serum), and have higher sensitivity and specificity. They are standardized and easily interpreted, but require specialized personnel to perform them [21].

2.2 Interpretation of the diagnostic tests

The gold standard in detecting viral infection is RT-PCR since its diagnostic precision is superior to the tests that detect the presence of the viral capsid antigens. SARS-CoV-2 antibody tests do not predict viral shedding and cannot be used to rule out risk of transmission. Rapid tests, both for antigens and antibodies, should be used for screening purposes only when (1) monitoring progression of a known positive case, or (2) when there is a very low suspicion of disease.

The presence of antibodies in COVID-19 patients should always be interpreted taking into account the result of the RT-PCR and the clinical phase of the disease. The levels of IgM and IgG antibodies could indicate host response to the virus [22].

Antibody seroprevalence levels of the general population – of those who have not suffered from the disease, or those who have only experienced its mild forms, – are needed in order to ascertain the significance of the antibodies, if the immune response is really protective, and how long this protection lasts [17].

2.3 Transmissibility and completion of isolation

The duration of transmissibility varies among patients with nondetectable, asymptomatic, mild, and severe symptoms. In general, there is evidence that virus transmission does not occur after the ninth asymptomatic day [23], although in severe cases, this point can be difficult to establish as residual symptoms may last longer.

In the general population, a negative RT-PCR is not considered sufficient to rule out transmissibility and the patient may require continued quarantine. The lack of replicable viral genetic material in the nasopharynx is a good indicator but not an absolute marker against transmissibility [24]. In asymptomatic patients isolated at home, the confinement may be terminated 10 days after a negative RT-PCR test. In symptomatic patients, the duration of the confinement should be 10 days from the resolution of symptoms including fever. Patients with severe or life-threatening symptoms may require an isolation duration of 21 days. The recommendations for healthcare personnel are different and at least one diagnostic test – either IgG or RT-PCR - should be performed prior to the end of the isolation period [15].

2.4 General screening of ENT patients who are candidates for surgery or invasive upper airway exploration

During the pandemic, head and neck clinicians should screen for active SARS-CoV-2 infection in all patients who are to undergo consultation, invasive examination, or ENT surgery. The choice of tests may vary according to the scale of coordinated response published by the region's healthcare governing body such as the Ministry of Health and Consumption and Social Welfare of the Government of Spain (MSCBS) [25].

Pre-operative screening should be performed by health or social-health personnel to all patients sufficiently in advance and, when possible, without face-to-face contact. The microbiological and immunological screening should entail RT-PCR ideally within 72 hours of procedure, followed by patient isolation to prevent subsequent infection. The screening should not be based on antigen testing [12].

Specific screening protocols depend on the specific alert scenario of the territory. In Spain, the following was recommended for the screening of active infections:

1. In Alert Level 2 or higher scenarios with unfavorable epidemiology, complete pre-surgical screening should be performed since both the patient and surgery are considered high risk (**Table 1**) (**Figure 1**).

2. If the epidemiology of the health area or territory is favorable (Alert Level 1), and with intermediate patient and surgery risks, RT-PCR could be replaced with "rapid" antigen testing (**Table 1**) (**Figure 2**).

3. If the epidemiology of the health area or territory is favorable (Alert Level 1), and with intermediate patient risk and low risk surgery, screening may be simplified (**Table 1**) (**Figure 2**).

In cases where surgery has been suspended, patients should be re-considered for surgery based on an asymptomatic period of at least 10 days. If symptoms or other suspicions persist, a repeat test should be undertaken within 72 hours prior to surgery. Both inpatients as well as outpatients scheduled for elective surgery should follow the same screening process and undergo repeat testing as indicated whether or not it was performed previously.

Additionally, patients with documented resolved infection in the last 3 months with an absence of symptoms and Alert Level 1 or lower epidemiology of the area likely do not require repeat RT-PCR testing. Nonetheless, the surgeon should review all risks and consider a delay of up to 4 weeks from the onset of symptoms [15].

The exact risks of treating vaccinated patients have not yet been well established. At this time, the authors recommend that all patients be treated with the same basic precautions afforded the non-immunized patients until further data becomes available.

2.5 Non-surgical protection measures for otolaryngologists and head and neck surgeons

The use of Personal Protective Equipment (PPE) should be mandatory regardless of the regional epidemiology until normality of care is reintroduced. Along with the basic precautions including appropriate work attire and disposable surgical masks, three degrees of precautions against airborne transmission have been defined [26] (**Table 2**).

Indicators		Estimate	Risk assessment				
			New normality	Low	Medium	High	Very high
BLOCK I: Evaluation of the transmission level.							
T1	Cumulative incidence of cases diagnosed in 14 days.	Confirmed cases (by diagnosis date) in 14 days *100,000/number of inhabitants.	≤25	>25 to ≤50	>50 to ≤150	>150 to ≤250	>250
T1'	Cumulative incidence of cases diagnosed in 7 days.	Confirmed cases (by diagnosis date) in 7 days *100,000/number of inhabitants.	≤10	>10 to ≤25	>25 to ≤75	>75 to ≤125	>125
T2	Cumulative incidence of cases aged ≥ 65 years diagnosed in 14 days.	Confirmed cases ≥ 65 years (by date of diagnosis) in 14 days *100,000/number of inhabitants > 65 years.	≤20	>20 to ≤50	>50 to ≤100	>100 to ≤150	>150
T2'	Cumulative incidence of cases aged ≥ 65 years diagnosed in 7 days.	Confirmed cases ≥ 65 years (by date of diagnosis) in 7 days *100,000/number of inhabitants ≥ 65 years.	≤10	>10 to ≤25	>25 to ≤50	>50 to ≤75	>75
T3	Global positivity of diagnostic tests for active infection (PDIA) per week.	N° of tests with a positive result in 7 days *100/N° of tests carried out in 7 days.	≤4%	>4% to ≤7%	>7% to ≤10%	>10% to ≤15%	>15%
T4	Percentage of cases with traceability.	N° of cases diagnosed with traceability *100/Total N° of confirmed cases diagnosed in the last 7 days.	>80%	≤80% to >65%	≤65% to >50	≤50% to >30%	≤30%
BLOCK II: Level of use of healthcare services due to COVID-19							
A1	Occupancy of hospital beds due to COVID-19 cases	N° of hospital beds occupied by COVID cases/Total hospital beds in operation.	≤2%	>2% to ≤5%	>5% to ≤10%	>10% to ≤15%	>15%
A2	Occupancy of critical care beds due to COVID-19 cases	N° of critical care beds occupied by COVID cases/Total N° of total critical care beds in operation.	≤5%	>5% to ≤10%	>10% to ≤15%	>15% to ≤25%	>25%

Table 1.
Indicators for risk assessment for COVID-19 [25]. Alert level 1: When at least two indicators from Block I and one from Block II are low; alert level 2: When at least two indicators from Block I and one from Block II are at medium level; alert level 3: When at least two indicators from Block I and one from Block II are at a high level; alert level 4: When at least two indicators from Block I and one from Block II are at a very high level.

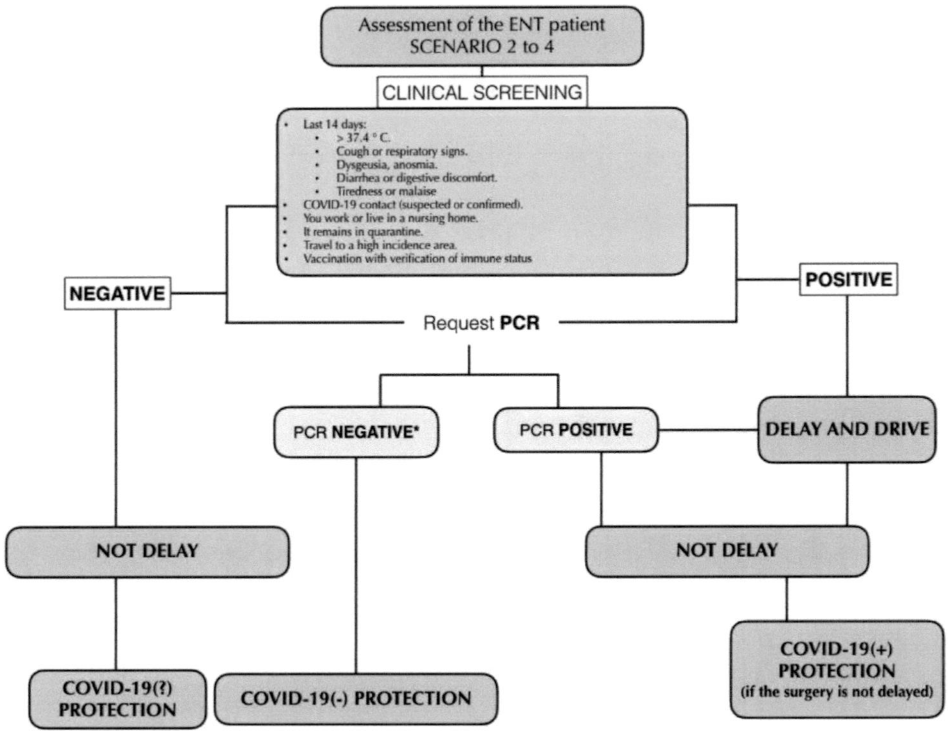

Figure 1.
Screening of the ENT patient at alert levels 2 or higher of the COVID-19 pandemic.

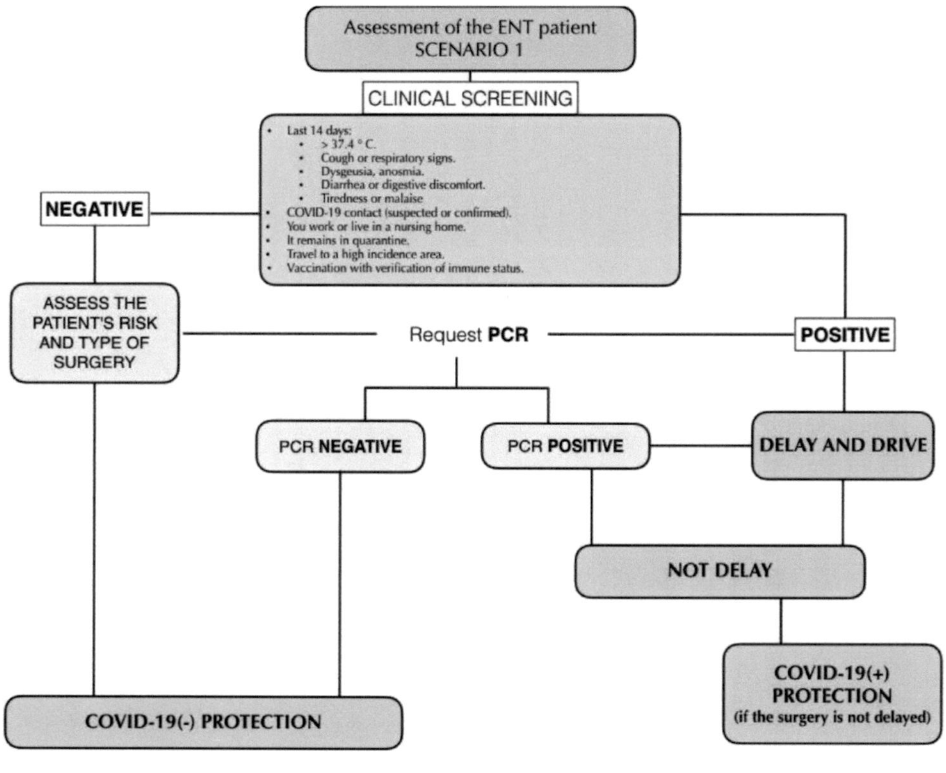

Figure 2.
Screening of the ENT patient at alert level 1 or lower during the COVID-19 pandemic.

	Grade 1	Grade 2	Grade 3
Workwear	Disposable medical uniform	Disposable medical uniform	Disposable medical uniform
Head protection	Waterproof medical cap	Waterproof medical cap	Waterproof medical cap
Mask	Surgical mask	N95/FFP2	FFP3
Protective coat	Not isolating	Isolation gown	Isolation gown
Gloves	Latex or equivalent.	Latex or equivalent	Latex or equivalent
Footwear	Not covered	Covered	Covered
Eye protection	—	Glasses. Screens	Glasses. Secreens
Motorized air purifying respirators	—	—	+

Table 2.
Individual precautions depending on the gradation of the risk of contagion [27].

In patients with hearing loss, tspecialized masks for lip reading can be used as long as there are no undo risks for the healthcare professional, such as the production of excess aerosols. [28, 29]. Hand washing and disinfection with hydroalcoholic gels should be conducted consistently based on WHO recommendations. [30, 31].

Relevant information regarding treatment policies should be accessible. Such information could be displayed either physically (posters, brochures, etc.) or online (websites and apps). They should include patient and provider expections such as the use of face-masks, social distancing, and hand hygiene [32], as well as infographics on loud verbalizations which could produce large amounts of projectile aerosols [33]. These spaces must be adapted with hydroalcoholic solution dispensers, waste containers with pedal-operated lid, as well as properly separated and indicated seats that help maintain a safe distance between people.

Waiting rooms should be modified so that patients are able to keep 2 meters between them (**Figure 3**). If the structure of the rooms make social distancing difficult, multiple waiting areas should be made available such that each area houses no more than three patients and companions.

Telemedicine is recommended whenever possible as it allows for safe consultation and helps prevent delays in care [34]. If the patient requires a face-to-face consultation, a prior clinical screening (preferably conducted remotely) is recommended. Again, waiting rooms should be modified so that patients can keep a distance 2 meters. Unnecessary fixtures and decorations should also be eliminated from the consultation area to facilitate movement of patients as well as medical equipment and to aid in subsequent disinfection [12, 26]. During consultation the door must remain closed with the air circulation for at least 15 minutes after each consult, especially at Alert Levels 2 or higher. HEPA (High Efficiency Particulate Air) filters, capable of filtering at least 99.97% of particles with a diameter greater than or equal to 0.3 μm in one cycle, should be utilized during disinfection of the consultation spaces [35].

The use of 0.5% povidone-iodine (PVP-I) in oral rinses and nasal drops could be used to decrease the local concentrations of the virus [36, 37], although there is no definite evidence that this measure reduces transmissibility and can lead to a false sense of security [38].

Specific precautionary measures have been outlined for non-surgical procedures in ENT in consultation and during hospital admission to the ward (**Table 3**).

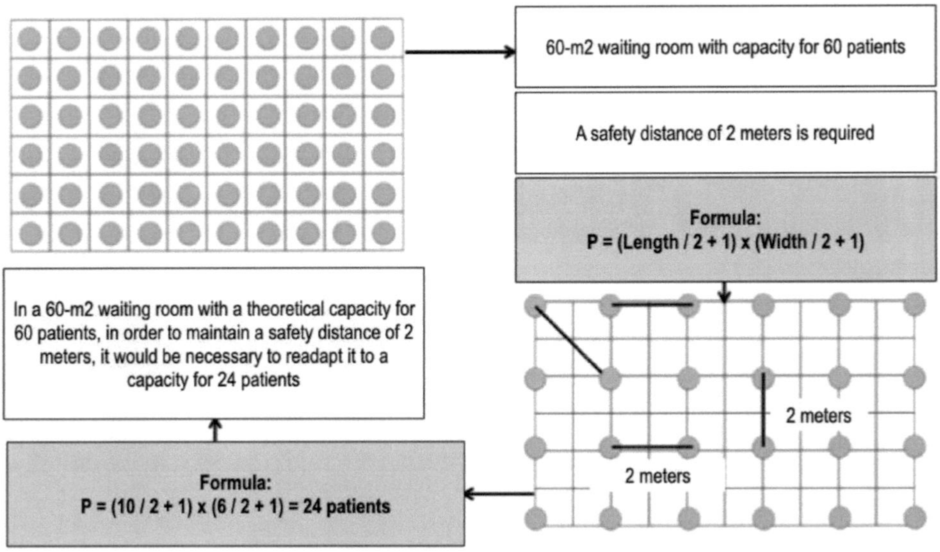

Figure 3.
Adaptation of the waiting room respecting a safety distance of 2 meters.

Audiometry tests are conducted in closed spaces that may be difficult to disinfect. Additional precautions must be taken during these examinations. Both the patient and the auxiliary personnel must each enter with a mask and should protect the surfaces they touch with proper hand hygiene and glove usage. The patient should be instructed to avoid touching surfaces other than the chair, and the tests themselves should be done via recording (**Table 4**).

Once the patient departs, the disposable materials must be disposed in their respective recepticles, and the contact surfaces disinfected using disposable antimicrobial cleaners. Many common cleaning and disinfection products are effective against coronaviruses, which can otherwise remain active on plastic and stainless steel surfaces for 2–3 days [50] and up to 9 days on other non-porous surfaces [35]. Among the most used cleaning agents are 0.1% sodium hypochlorite solution, hydroalcoholic solution, and ethanol solution (concentration of 62–71%) [43]. While direct investigations have not yet been conducted, studies in similar coronoviruses have suggested an effective eradication time after approximately 1 minute of contact [35].

Ultraviolet light (UV-C) may provide another method of sterilization even when used to decontaminate porous surfaces like masks [51]. In fact, the most efficient sterilization may entail a combination of both chemical and UV-C exposure [52]. The Spanish Society for Environmental Health (SESA) advises against the use of chlorine dioxide for atmospheric disinfection. Similarly, ozone disinfection requires a high concentration which poses risks of toxicity, requiring extended periods of evacuation.

3. Specific and transversal surgical measures

The prevention measures executed by the surgical team are carried out with the aim of protecting the team as well as the patient. The nasopharynx retains a relatively high viral load, and procedures in this area are associated with aerosolization and dissemination of viral particles particularly during the use of drills,

Procedure	Recommendation
Rigid or flexible endoscopy	• Use of tower with camera and screen to increase the distance between the patient and the examiner as much as possible.. • Prevent the patient from removing the mask, but have them lower it partially. As an alternative, the clinician may use a system that seals the nose during examination.(**Figure 4**) [12, 39]. • Avoid unnecessary endonasal manipulations. • Replace aerosol local anesthetics with those applied using cotton wicks or lenses [40, 41]. • Resorbable nasal packs should be used for acute or postsurgical epistaxis [11, 42]. • The removal of a nasal packing should be carried out after appropriate equipment measurements according to the classification of the patient (**Table 2**). • Disinfection with phenolic compounds, peracetic acid, or sodium hypochlorite is prudent. As an alternative, protective covers should be utilized [43].
Otomicroscope	• Disposable materials should be used whenever applicable. • Barriers should be placed between the microscope and the patient such as methacrylate screens adapted to the binocular or disposable plastic covers (**Figure 5**). • After examination, patient contact areas must be cleaned and disinfected [12, 44].
Vestibular tests	• General consultation and audiometry recommendations should be followed (**Table 4**).
Hearing Screening for Newborns	• Each screening should be conducted by personnel who do not work directly with COVID19 patients, especially if the mother is asymptomatic. • General patient PPEs should be utilized in all cases, and specific protections can be escalated according to the degree of contagion risk (**Table 2**). • The equipment must be decontaminated after each use. • There are some indications that children born during the COVID-19 pandemic should be retested at the conclusion of the pandemic [45].
Post-tracheostomy care	• In patients with confirmed infection, tracheostomy cuffs should remain inflated. In-line suction systems should be utilized and tracheostomy tube changes should be delayed until the RT-PCR becomes negative. [46, 47]. • High risk aerosol precautions should be followed even in asymptomatic patients.
CPAP or BiPAP devices for obstructive sleep apnea syndrome (OSA):	• Incomplete seals around the face may facilitate the risk of aerosol generation. • The use of helmet-type CPAP masks is recommended to reduce the risk of transmission [48, 49].

Table 3.
Specific precautionary measures during non-surgical procedures in ENT in consultation and during hospital admission to the ward.

microdebridators, and/or electric or ultrasonic scalpels [11, 48, 53–55]. All patients planned for aerodigestive tract surgery should be screened according to the Alert Level of the pandemic (**Figures 1** and **2**). A consent form detailing the risks and

	Contagious status and severity of hearing loss		
	COVID-19 (−)	COVID-19 (?) or COVID-19 (+)	
Technical and material indication		**Suspicion of sudden hearing loss**	**Without suspicion of sudden hearing loss**
Single act or delay audiometry	Perform audiometry on the spot (prior written or oral explanation facilitating the patient's lip reading)		Delay Treatment
Use of soundproof booth	Yes	According to clinical criteria (will be noted in the HC if the cabin is not used)	
Protection of the patient's face, head and hands	Surgical mask	FFP2/KN95/N95, disposable cap, hand washing and gloves	
Headphone protection	Protect the earpiece and vibrator with disposable material (preferably use single-use insert earphones)		
Positive response indication	Raising a hand, without using the push button		
Stimulation in speech audiometry	Use recording		
Cleaning after finishing the test	1) audiometer, 2) patient chair, 3) earpiece, 4) vibrator, 5) clean and air the cabin if used		

Table 4.
Carrying out audiometry; indications and protective measures for the clinician and the patient. COVID-19 (−): Case ruled out/COVID-19 (?): Probable or suspected case/COVID-19 (+): Confirmed case [12].

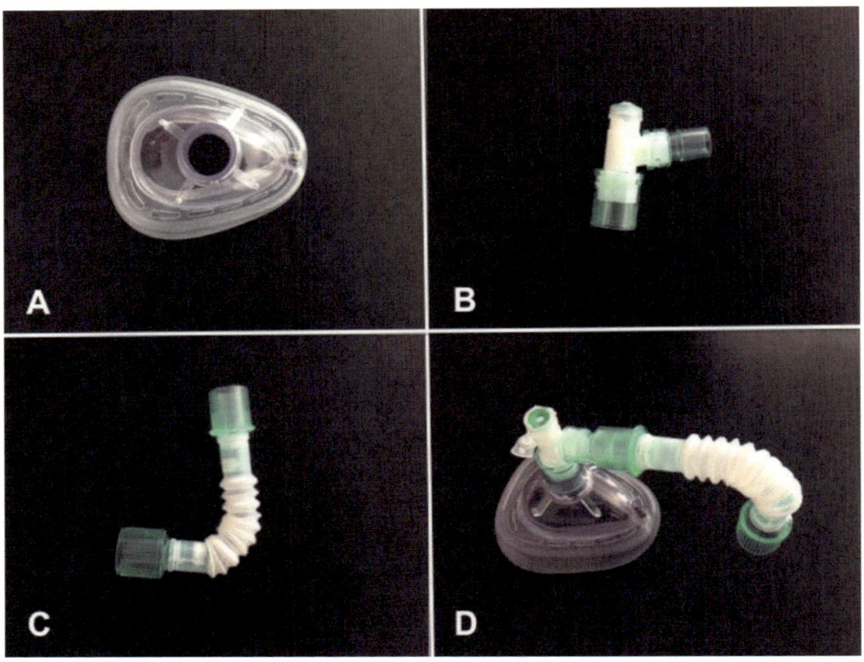

Figure 4.
Nasal fibroendoscopy examination system. (A) Anesthesia mask. (B) Connection piece with a valve used to introduce the nasofibrolaryngoscope. (C) Tubing to direct the patient's air away from the examiner. (D) Proper assembly.

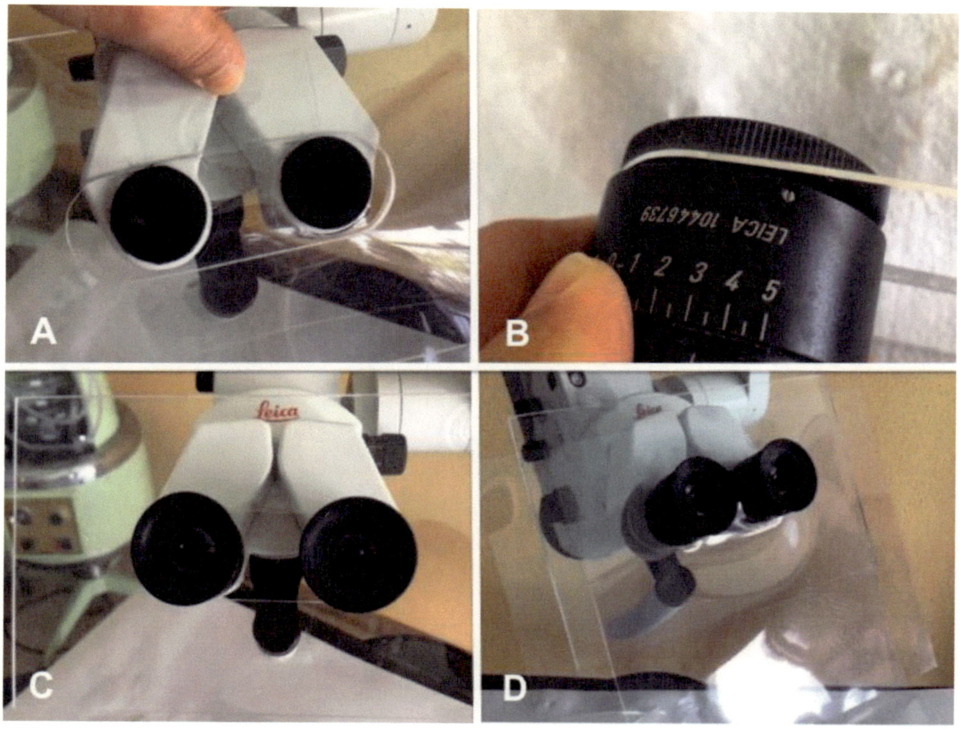

Figure 5.
Microscope examination system (A) Methacrylate screen adapted to the microscope after removing the eye pieces. (B) Adaptation of the eye pieces to the slotted screen that allows manipulation of the interpupillary distance. (C) Adaptation of the eye pieces to the microscope with the methacrylate screen in place. (D) Interposed and replaceable plastic screens to improve sealing.

protective measures should also be presented [56], During the Alert Level 4, all elective surgery should be postponed [57]. Considering the large numbers of asymptomatic COVID cases, all patients without evidence to the contrary should be assumed as positive for SARS-CoV-2 and the appropriate protective measures should be taken [57].

A negative pressure surgical environment is recommended via a high frequency of air cirulation (25 circuits per hour) that reduces the viral load inside the operating room [58]. The same operating room and non-disposable anesthesia equipment is recommended for all probable or confirmed COVID-19 patients [58, 59]. This includes urgent cases in which SARS-CoV-2 infection has not been ruled out. Likewise, during Alerts Level 2 or higher, the number of surgical team members should also be limited [41]. Endotracheal intubation and air-purifying respirators should be used at the time of induction [60] and the anesthesia must be sufficiently deep to avoid intraoperative awakening or coughing. The use of a closed suction system with an antiviral filter is recommended [61].

Aerosolized particles of less than 5 μm can remain in suspension for more than 3 hours, so the use of instruments that generate aerosols or particles in suspension (microdebriders, high-speed motors, electric or ultrasonic scalpels) should be avoided whenever possible [50].

Individual protection measures will be adapted according to the classification of the patient (**Table 5**). In the immediate postoperative period, and once an Alert Level 2 or higher is established, communication with the family members should be conducted electronically [72].

Surgical individual protection measures			
	Infectious status of the patient		
Anatomic area to protect	**COVID-19 (−)**	**COVID-19 (?)**	**COVID-19 (+)**
Feet	Work shoes (clogs) with disposable footwear	Work shoes (clogs) with double disposable gaiter	
Body (Trunk and extremities, except feet and hands)	Medical uniform + non-waterproof disposable surgical gown	Medical uniform + waterproof surgical gown	Medical uniform + impermeable seals between PPE components + waterproof surgical gown
Head (Scalp, pinna and external auditory canal)	Disposable surgical cap	Double sterile surgical cap	
Hands	Simple sterile surgical glove	Double sterile surgical glove	
Face and neck (Forehead, neck, periauricular region)	Face shield (optional)	Face shield	Full face protective helmet or powered air-purifying respirators
Eyes	Non-integral glasses	Integral glasses	Face shield + sealing goggles + impermeable covers for the forehead, neck, and chest
Respiratory (Mouth, nostrils and external auditory canal)	Surgical mask	FFP3	FFP3
Specific measures during surgical or invasive procedures in ENT (Alert levels 2 or higher)			
Airway management and diagnostic airway procedures (excluding tracheostomy) [62]	• Performed by the physician with the most experience in rapid sequence intubation techniques. • Disposable laryngoscopes and video laryngoscopes. • Avoid intubations with fiber optics. • Perform airway procedures for patients with suspected, probable, or positive COVID-19 status with endotracheal intubation. • Minimize spontaneous ventilation and repeated intubation/extubation.		
Tracheostomy	• Emergency tracheostomy confers a significant risk of aerosolization of the virus and should be proceeded with extreme caution [60]. • Delay elective tracheostomy, if possible, until the infected patient becomes negative. • COVID-19 (+) tracheostomy patients should be kept in a closed circuit with inline suction. • Delay cannula changes whenever possible until the infection resolves. If it is necessary to perform in a negative pressure room with HEPA filtration and an improved PPE, diver type, must be used for all personnel [46, 47].		

Surgical individual protection measures			
	Infectious status of the patient		
Anatomic area to protect	**COVID-19 (−)**	**COVID-19 (?)**	**COVID-19 (+)**
Oral cavity, oropharynx, nasal cavity and nasopharynx procedures	• Postpone elective procedures involving the nasal cavity, nasopharynx, oral cavity and oropharynx in suspected, probable or positive patients until negative [48]. • In order to avoid admissions for post-tonsillectomy bleeding, utilize techniques with lowest risks of postoperative complications including bleeding (intracapsular tonsillectomy) [45, 63].		
Otologic surgery	• As the presence of the virus in otitis media with effusion is not ruled out [64], procedures such as transtympanic drains should be avoided [45, 65]. • Mastoidectomy should be postponed whenever possible. If mastoidectomy is required, PPE should be worn and high-speed motors should be avoided [66].		
Endoscopic sinonasal surgery [67, 68]	• Avoid the use of microdebriders, high resolution motors, or surgical drills whenever possible. • In case it is not possible to delay an anterior skull base intervention in a COVID-19 (+) patient, a transcranial approach could be considered in order to avoid sinonasal surgery, which presents a much higher risk of virus aerosolization [69]. The degree of viral involvement inf brain tissue, although suspected [70], appears to be much lower that of sinonasal tissues. • Use resorbable tamponades postoperatively.		
Surgery of the head and neck, and of the deep cervical spaces [71, 72]	• Postpone surgical excision of benign neck masses during Alert levels 2 or higher. • Pediatric cases with solid head and neck tumors including thyroid cancer should be discussed in a multidisciplinary tumor Commission to decide the most appropriate treatment modality, taking into account the availability of local resources. • Head and neck cancer patients who require surgical treatment, who have been proposed for this purpose in the relevant Commission, will have priority over other non-cancer procedures, regardless of the Alert Level of the pandemic. • Whenever possible, medical treatment of infectious diseases should be attempted prior to surgical intervention.		

Table 5.
Professional protection measures in the operating room and during high risk procedures outside the operating room. COVID-19 (−): Case ruled out/ COVID-19 (?): Probable or suspected case/ COVID-19 (+): Confirmed case.

Author details

Juan Manuel Maza-Solano[1], Antonio Jiménez-Luna[2], Pablo Parente-Arias[3], Juan Carlos Amor-Dorado[4], Christian Calvo-Henriquez[5] and Guillermo Plaza-Mayor[6]*

1 Otolaryngology Department, Hospital Universitario Virgen Macarena, Hospital Quirónsalud Sagrado Corazón, Sevilla, Spain

2 Otolaryngology Department, Agencia Sanitaria Alto Guadalquivir (Hospital Valle del Guadiato y Hospital de Puente Genil), Hospital Quirónsalud de Córdoba, Córdoba, Spain

3 Otolaryngology Department, Hospital Universitario Lucus Augusti, Lugo, Spain

4 Otolaryngology Department, Hospital Can Misses, Ibiza, Spain

5 Otolaryngology Department, Hospital Universitario Santiago de Compostela, Coruña, Spain

6 Otolaryngology Department, Hospital Universitario de Fuenlabrada, Universidad Rey Juan Carlos, Madrid, Spain

*Address all correspondence to: guillermo.plaza@salud.madrid.org

References

[1] Zhou P, Yang X-L, Wang X-G, Hu B, Zhang L, Zhang W, et al. A pneumonia outbreak associated with a new coronavirus of probable bat origin. Nature. 2020 Mar;579(7798):270-3.

[2] Lu R, Zhao X, Li J, Niu P, Yang B, Wu H, et al. Genomic characterisation and epidemiology of 2019 novel coronavirus: implications for virus origins and receptor binding. Lancet. 2020 Feb 22;395(10224):565-74.

[3] Koh WC, Naing L, Chaw L, Rosledzana MA, Alikhan MF, Jamaludin SA, et al. What do we know about SARS-CoV-2 transmission? A systematic review and meta-analysis of the secondary attack rate and associated risk factors. PloS One. 2020;15(10):e0240205.

[4] Bax A, Bax CE, Stadnytskyi V, Anfinrud P. SARS-CoV-2 transmission via speech-generated respiratory droplets. Lancet Infect Dis. 2021 Mar;21(3):318.

[5] Wassie GT, Azene AG, Bantie GM, Dessie G, Aragaw AM. Incubation Period of Severe Acute Respiratory Syndrome Novel Coronavirus 2 that Causes Coronavirus Disease 2019: A Systematic Review and Meta-Analysis. Curr Ther Res Clin Exp. 2020;93:100607.

[6] He J, Guo Y, Mao R, Zhang J. Proportion of asymptomatic coronavirus disease 2019: A systematic review and meta-analysis. J Med Virol. 2021 Feb;93(2):820-30.

[7] Meyerowitz-Katz G, Merone L. A systematic review and meta-analysis of published research data on COVID-19 infection fatality rates. Int J Infect Dis IJID Off Publ Int Soc Infect Dis. 2020 Dec;101:138-48.

[8] Levin AT, Hanage WP, Owusu-Boaitey N, Cochran KB, Walsh SP, Meyerowitz-Katz G. Assessing the age specificity of infection fatality rates for COVID-19: systematic review, meta-analysis, and public policy implications. Eur J Epidemiol. 2020 Dec;35(12):1123-38.

[9] Sayampanathan AA, Heng CS, Pin PH, Pang J, Leong TY, Lee VJ. Infectivity of asymptomatic versus symptomatic COVID-19. Lancet Lond Engl. 2021 Jan 9;397(10269):93-4.

[10] Sahu AK, Amrithanand VT, Mathew R, Aggarwal P, Nayer J, Bhoi S. COVID-19 in health care workers - A systematic review and meta-analysis. Am J Emerg Med. 2020 Sep;38(9):1727-31.

[11] Workman AD, Welling DB, Carter BS, Curry WT, Holbrook EH, Gray ST, et al. Endonasal instrumentation and aerosolization risk in the era of COVID-19: simulation, literature review, and proposed mitigation strategies. Int Forum Allergy Rhinol. 2020 Sep;163(3):465-470.

[12] Maza-Solano JM, Plaza-Mayor G, Jiménez-Luna A, Parente-Arias P, Amor-Dorado JC. Strategies for the Practice of Otolaryngology and Head and Neck Surgery During the Monitoring Phase of COVID-19. Acta Otorrinolaringol Esp. 2020;71(6):367-78.

[13] Martin-Villares C, Bernal-Sprekelsen M, Molina-Ramirez CP, Bartolome-Benito M. Risk of contagion of SARS-CoV-2 among otorhinolaryngologists in Spain during the "Two waves". Eur Arch Otorhinolaryngol. 2021 Sep;278(9):3571-3577.

[14] Actuaciones de respuesta coordinada para el control de la transmisión de COVID-19 In: Sanidad Md, editor. 2020 [Internet]. [Internet]. [cited 2021 Jan 31]. Available from: https://www.mscbs.gob.es/profesionales/saludPublica/ccayes/alertasActual/nCov/documentos/

Actuaciones_respuesta_COVID_22.10.2020.pdf

[15] Estrategia de detección precoz, vigilancia y control de COVID-19. In: Sanidad Md, editor. 2020. [Internet] [Internet]. 2020 [cited 2021 Feb 15]. Available from: https://www.mscbs.gob.es/profesionales/saludPublica/ccayes/alertasActual/nCov/documentos/COVID19_Estrategia_vigilancia_y_control_e_indicadores.pdf

[16] Wölfel R, Corman VM, Guggemos W, Seilmaier M, Zange S, Müller MA, et al. Virological assessment of hospitalized patients with COVID-2019. Nature [Internet]. 2020 Apr 1; Available from: https://doi.org/10.1038/s41586-020-2196-x

[17] Altmann DM, Douek DC, Boyton RJ. What policy makers need to know about COVID-19 protective immunity. Lancet. 2020 May 16;395(10236):1527-1529.

[18] Wu F, Wang A, Liu M, Wang Q, Chen J, Xia S, et al. Neutralizing antibody responses to SARS-CoV-2 in a COVID-19 recovered patient cohort and their implications. medRxiv. 2020 Jan 1;2020.03.30.20047365.

[19] Tan W, Lu Y, Zhang J, Wang J, Dan Y, Tan Z, et al. Viral Kinetics and Antibody Responses in Patients with COVID-19. medRxiv. 2020 Jan 1;2020.03.24.20042382.

[20] Zhao J, Yuan Q, Wang H, Liu W, Liao X, Su Y, et al. Antibody responses to SARS-CoV-2 in patients of novel coronavirus disease 2019. Clin Infect Dis. 2020 Nov 19;71(16):2027-2034.

[21] Grupo de expertos SEIMC para el análisis del diagnóstico microbiológico del COVID-19. Recomendaciones institucionales. Documento de posicionamiento de la SEIMC sobre el diagnóstico microbiológico de COVID-19 [Internet]. [cited 2021 Feb 15]. Available from: https://seimc.org/contenidos/documentoscientificos/recomendaciones/seimc-rc-2020-Posicionamiento_SEIMC_diagnostico_microbiologico_COVID19.pdf

[22] Petherick A. Developing antibody tests for SARS-CoV-2. Lancet Lond Engl. 2020 Apr 4;395(10230):1101-2.

[23] Cevik M, Tate M, Lloyd O, Maraolo AE, Schafers J, Ho A. SARS-CoV-2, SARS-CoV, and MERS-CoV viral load dynamics, duration of viral shedding, and infectiousness: a systematic review and meta-analysis. Lancet Microbe. 2021 Jan 1;2(1):e13-22.

[24] European Centre for Disease Prevention and Control. Guidance for discharge and ending isolation of people with COVID-19, 16 October 2020. Stockholm: ECDC; 2020.

[25] Actuaciones de respuesta coordinada para el control de la transmisión de COVID-19 In: Sanidad Md, editor. 2020.

[26] Zou L, Ruan F, Huang M, Liang L, Huang H, Hong Z, et al. SARS-CoV-2 Viral Load in Upper Respiratory Specimens of Infected Patients. N Engl J Med. 2020 Feb 19;382(12):1177-9.

[27] Liu Z, Zhang L. At the center of the COVID-19 pandemic: Lessons learned for otolaryngology-head and neck surgery in China. Int Forum Allergy Rhinol. 2020 May;10(5):584-6.

[28] Brücher BLDM, Nigri G, Tinelli A, Lapeña JFF, Espin-Basany E, Macri P, et al. COVID-19: Pandemic surgery guidance. 4open [Internet]. 2020;3. Available from: https://doi.org/10.1051/fopen/2020002

[29] Bartoszko JJ, Farooqi MAM, Alhazzani W, Loeb M. Medical masks vs N95 respirators for preventing COVID-19 in healthcare workers: A systematic review and meta-analysis of randomized trials. Influenza Other Respir Viruses. 2020 Jul;14(4):365-373.

[30] WHO. Sus 5 momentos para la higiene de manos. [Internet]. [cited 2021 Jan 31]. Available from: https://www.who.int/gpsc/information_centre/gpsc_5_momentos_poster_es.pdf?ua=1

[31] WHO. La higiene de manos y el recorrido del paciente quirúrgico. [Internet]. [cited 2021 Jan 31]. Available from: https://www.who.int/gpsc/5may/hh_infographic_A3_ES.pdf?ua=1

[32] Documento técnico. Manejo en atención primaria y domiciliaria del COVID-19 [Internet]. [Internet]. 2020 [cited 2021 Jan 28]. Available from: https://www.mscbs.gob.es/profesionales/saludPublica/ccayes/alertasActual/nCov-China/documentos/Manejo_primaria.pdf

[33] Asadi S, Wexler AS, Cappa CD, Barreda S, Bouvier NM, Ristenpart WD. Aerosol emission and superemission during human speech increase with voice loudness. Sci Rep. 2019 Feb 20;9(1):2348.

[34] Ning AY, Cabrera CI, D'Anza B. Telemedicine in Otolaryngology: A Systematic Review of Image Quality, Diagnostic Concordance, and Patient and Provider Satisfaction. Ann Otol Rhinol Laryngol. 2021 Feb;130(2):195-204.

[35] Kampf G, Todt D, Pfaender S, Steinmann E. Persistence of coronaviruses on inanimate surfaces and their inactivation with biocidal agents. J Hosp Infect. 2020 Mar 1;104(3):246-51.

[36] Khan MM, Parab SR. 0.5% povidone iodine irrigation in otorhinolaryngology surgical practice during COVID 19 pandemic. Am J Otolaryngol. 2020 Dec;41(6):102687.

[37] Frank S, Capriotti J, Brown SM, Tessema B. Povidone-Iodine Use in Sinonasal and Oral Cavities: A Review of Safety in the. Ear Nose Throat J. 2020 Nov;99(9):586-93.

[38] Burton MJ, Clarkson JE, Goulao B, Glenny A-M, McBain AJ, Schilder AGM, Webster KE, Worthington HV. Antimicrobial mouthwashes (gargling) and nasal sprays administered to patients with suspected or confirmed COVID-19 infection to improve patient outcomes and to protect healthcare workers treating them. Cochrane Database of Systematic Reviews 2020, Issue 9. Art. No.: CD013627. DOI: 10.1002/14651858.CD013627.pub2.

[39] Lechien JR, Chiesa-Estomba CM, De Siati DR, Horoi M, Le Bon SD, Rodriguez A, et al. Olfactory and gustatory dysfunctions as a clinical presentation of mild-to-moderate forms of the coronavirus disease (COVID-19): a multicenter European study. Eur Arch Otorhinolaryngol [Internet]. 2020 Apr 6; Available from: https://doi.org/10.1007/s00405-020-05965-1

[40] Kamming D, Gardam M, Chung F. Anaesthesia and SARS. Br J Anaesth. 2003 Jun;90(6):715-8.

[41] Van Gerven L, Hellings PW, Cox T, Fokkens W, Hopkins C, Hox V, et al. Personal protection and delivery of rhinologic and endoscopic skull base procedures during the COVID-19 Rhinology. 2020 Jun 1;58(3):289-294.

[42] Workman AD, Jafari A, Welling DB, Varvares MA, Gray ST, Holbrook EH, et al. Airborne Aerosol Generation During Endonasal Procedures in the Era of COVID-19: Risks and Recommendations. Otolaryngol Neck Surg. 2020 May 26;163(3):465-70.

[43] List N: Disinfectants for Use Against SARS-CoV-2 [Internet]. 2020 [cited 2021 Jul 2]. Available from: List N: Disinfectants for Use Against SARS-CoV-2. United States Environmental Protection Agency. https://www.epa.gov/ pesticide-registration/list-n-disinfectants-useagainst-sars-cov-2. Published 2020).

[44] Lavilla MJ, Huarte A, Cavallé L, Núñez F. Medidas de desinfección e

higiene en audiología y estrategias comunicativas durante pandemia COVID-19 [Internet]. [cited 2021 Feb 16]. Available from: https://seorl.net/wp-content/uploads/2020/04/MEDIDAS-DE-DESINFECCIÓN-E-HIGIENE-EN-AUDIOLOGÍA-Y-ESTRATEGIAS-COMUNICATIVAS-DURANTE-LA-PANDEMIA-COVID-19.pdf

[45] Leboulanger N, Sagardoy T, Akkari M, Ayari-Khalfallah S, Celerier C, Fayoux P, et al. COVID-19 and ENT Pediatric otolaryngology during the COVID-19 pandemic. Guidelines of the French Association of Pediatric Otorhinolaryngology (AFOP) and French Society of Otorhinolaryngology (SFORL). Eur Ann Otorhinolaryngol Head Neck Dis. 2020 May;137(3):177-81.

[46] Díaz de Cerio Canduela P, Ferrandis Perepérez E, Parente Arias P, López Álvarez F, Sistiaga Suarez JA. Recommendations of the Spanish Society of Otolaryngology and Head and Neck Surgery for performing tracheotomies in patients infected by the coronavirus, Covid-19. Acta Otorrinolaringol Esp. 2020 Aug;71(4):253-5.

[47] Martin-Villares C, Perez Molina-Ramirez C, Bartolome-Benito M, Bernal-Sprekelsen M. Outcome of 1890 tracheostomies for critical COVID-19 patients: a national cohort study in Spain. Eur Arch Otorhinolaryngol. 2021 May;278(5):1605-1612.

[48] Bann DV, Patel VA, Saadi R, Gniady JP, Goyal N, McGinn JD, et al. Impact of Coronavirus (COVID-19) on Otolaryngologic Surgery: A Brief Commentary. Head Neck. 2020 Apr 9;

[49] Tran K, Cimon K, Severn M, Pessoa-Silva CL, Conly J. Aerosol generating procedures and risk of transmission of acute respiratory infections to healthcare workers: a systematic review. PloS One. 2012;7(4): e35797.

[50] van Doremalen N, Bushmaker T, Morris DH, Holbrook MG, Gamble A, Williamson BN, et al. Aerosol and Surface Stability of SARS-CoV-2 as Compared with SARS-CoV-1. N Engl J Med. 2020 Mar 17;

[51] Hamzavi IH, Lyons AB, Kohli I, Narla S, Parks-Miller A, Gelfand JM, et al. Ultraviolet germicidal irradiation: possible method for respirator disinfection to facilitate reuse during COVID-19 pandemic. J Am Acad Dermatol. 2020 Apr 1;

[52] Dexter F, Parra MC, Brown JR, Loftus RW. Perioperative COVID-19 Defense: An Evidence-Based Approach for Optimization of Infection Control and Operating Room Management. Anesth Analg. 2020 Jul;131(1):37-42.

[53] Patel R, Babady E, Theel ES, Storch GA, Pinsky BA, St George K, et al. Report from the American Society for Microbiology COVID-19 International Summit, 23 March 2020: Value of Diagnostic Testing for SARS-CoV-2/COVID-19. mBio. 2020 Mar 26;11(2):e00722-20.

[54] Lauer SA, Grantz KH, Bi Q, Jones FK, Zheng Q, Meredith HR, et al. The Incubation Period of Coronavirus Disease 2019 (COVID-19) From Publicly Reported Confirmed Cases: Estimation and Application. Ann Intern Med. 2020 May 5;172(9):577-582.

[55] Wang J, Zhou M, Liu F. Reasons for healthcare workers becoming infected with novel coronavirus disease 2019 (COVID-19) in China. J Hosp Infect. 2020 May;105(1):100-101.

[56] Sociedad Española de Otorrinolaringología y Cirugía de Cabeza y Cuello (SEORLCCC). Documento de información y autorización para la realización de exploraciones e intervenciones quirúrgicas durante la pandemia por COVID-19 [Internet]. [cited 2021 Feb 15]. Available from:

https://seorl.net/wp-content/uploads/2020/05/documento-de-informacion-y-autorizacion-para-la-realizacion-de-exploraciones-e-intervenciones-qx-durante-la-pandemia-por-covid-19.pdf

[57] Somashekhar SP, Shivaram HV, Abhaham SJ, Dalvi A, Kumar A, Gode D, et al. ASI's Consensus Guidelines: ABCs of What to Do and What Not During the COVID-19 Pandemic. Indian J Surg. 2020 Jun 1;82(3):240-50.

[58] Kowalski LP, Sanabria A, Ridge JA, Ng WT, de Bree R, Rinaldo A, et al. COVID-19 pandemic: effects and evidence-based recommendations for otolaryngology and head and neck surgery practice. Head Neck. 2020 Jun;42(6):1259-1267.

[59] Ti LK, Ang LS, Foong TW, Ng BSW. What we do when a COVID-19 patient needs an operation: operating room preparation and guidance. Can J Anaesth. 2020 Jun;67(6):756-758.

[60] Wax RS, Christian MD. Practical recommendations for critical care and anesthesiology teams caring for novel coronavirus (2019-nCoV) patients. Can J Anaesth. 2020 May;67(5):568-576.

[61] Martín Delgado MC, Avilés-Jurado FX, Álvarez Escudero J, Aldecoa Álvarez-Santuyano C, de Haro López C, Díaz de Cerio Canduela P, et al. Consensus document of the Spanish Society of Intensive and Critical Care Medicine and Coronary Units (SEMICYUC), the Spanish Society of Otorhinolaryngology and Head and Neck Surgery (SEORL-CCC) and the Spanish Society of Anesthesiology and Resuscitation (SEDAR) on tracheotomy in patients with COVID-19 infection. Med Intensiva Engl Ed. 2020;44(8):493-9.

[62] Villalonga Vadell R, Martín Delgado MC, Avilés-Jurado FX, Álvarez Escudero J, Aldecoa Álvarez-Santuyano C, de Haro López C, et al. Consensus Document of the Spanish Society of Intensive and Critical Care Medicine and Coronary Units (SEMICYUC), the Spanish Society of Otorhinolaryngology and Head and Neck Surgery (SEORL-CCC) and the Spanish Society of Anesthesiology and Resuscitation (SEDAR) on Tracheotomy in Patients with COVID-19 Infection. Rev Esp Anestesiol Reanim. 2020 Nov;67(9):504-10.

[63] Comisión de Otorrinolaringología Pediátrica, Grupo de trabajo en COVID, Comisión delegada de la SEORLCCC. Recomendaciones en el manejo del paciente pediátrico en el contexto de la pandemia por COVID-19 [Internet]. [Internet]. [cited 2021 Jan 31]. Available from: https://seorl.net/wp-content/uploads/2020/03/RECOMENDACIONES-EN-EL-MANEJO-DEL-PACIENTE-PEDIÁTRICO-EN-EL-CONTEXTO-DE-LA-PANDEMIA-POR-COVID-19-1.pdf

[64] Maharaj S, Bello Alvarez M, Mungul S, Hari K. Otologic dysfunction in patients with COVID-19: A systematic review. Laryngoscope Investig Otolaryngol. 2020 Dec;5(6):1192-6.

[65] Chorney SR, Elden LM, Giordano T, Kazahaya K, Rizzi MD, Zur KB, et al. Algorithm-Based Pediatric Otolaryngology Management During the COVID-19 Global Pandemic: A Children's Hospital of Philadelphia Clinical Consensus. Otolaryngol Head Neck Surg. 2020 Jul;163(1):25-37.

[66] Markey AL, Leong SC, Vaughan C. Droplet and bone dust contamination from high-speed drilling during mastoidectomy. Clin Otolaryngol. 2021 May;46(3):614-618.

[67] Jones HAS, Salib RJ, Harries PG. Reducing Aerosolized Particles and Droplet Spread in Endoscopic Sinus Surgery during. Laryngoscope. 2021 May;131(5):956-960.

[68] Viera-Artiles J, Mato D, Valdiande JJ, Lobo D, Pedraja J, López-Higuera JM, et al. A novel aerosolisation mitigation device for endoscopic sinus and skull base surgery in the COVID-19 era. Eur Arch Otorhinolaryngol. 2021 Jun;278(6):1869-1877.

[69] Patel ZM, Fernandez-Miranda J, Hwang PH, Nayak JV, Dodd R, Sajjadi H, et al. Precautions for endoscopic transnasal skull base surgery during the COVID-19 pandemic. Neurosurgery. 2020 Jul 1;87(1):E66-E67.

[70] Kabbani N, Olds JL. Does COVID19 Infect the Brain? If So, Smokers Might Be at a Higher Risk. Mol Pharmacol. 2020 May;97(5):351-3.

[71] Bann DV, Patel VA, Saadi R, Goyal N, Gniady JP, McGinn JD, et al. Best Practice Recommendations for Pediatric Otolaryngology during the COVID-19 Pandemic. Otolaryngol Head Neck Surg. 2020 Jun;162(6):783-794.

[72] Prin M, Bartels K. Social distancing: implications for the operating room in the face of COVID-19. Can J Anaesth. 2020 Jul;67(7):789-797.